D1146731

Ageless Yoga

Aberdeenshire Library and Information Service
www.aberdeenshire.gov.uk/libraries
Renewals Hotline 01224 661511

HEADQUARTERS

1 2 MAY 2006

2 5 SEP 2006

2 7 NOV 2006

2 4 SEP 2007

2 7 AUG 2008

- 2 MAR 2011

29 MAR 2011

2 8 APR 2011

1 8 JUN 2011

1 6 JUL 2011

1 9 AUG 2011

- 1 OCT 2011

- 5 APR 2012

0 4 OCT 2012

- 6 NOV 2012

- 7 MAR 2014

0 2 NOV 2016

ABERDEENSHIRE
LIBRARIES
PEGRUM, Juliet
WITHDRAWN
FROM LIBRARY
Ageless yoga

A L I S
1714481

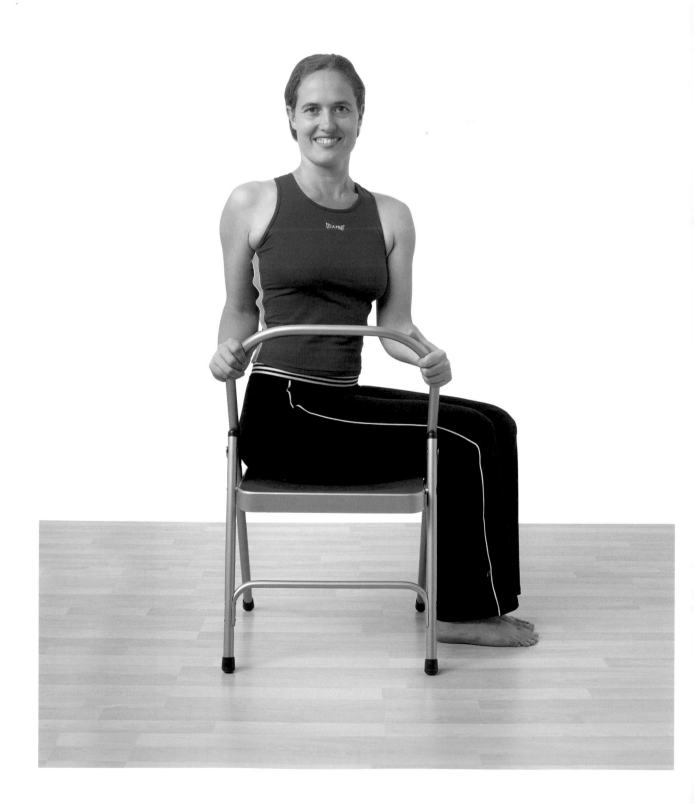

Ageless Yoga

Gentle Workouts
for Health & Fitness

JULIET PEGRUM

CICO BOOKS
London

AUTHOR'S ACKNOWLEDGMENTS

*To all my kind teachers who tirelessly share their wisdom and to all who seek happiness
and freedom through the practices of yoga.*

Juliet Pegrum can be contacted at: julietpegrum@mahamudrayoga.com

First published in 2006 by Cico Books Ltd
32 Great Sutton Street London EC1V 0NB
Copyright © Cico Books 2005

The right of Juliet Pegrum to be identified as author of this text has been asserted by
her in accordance with the Copyright, Designs and Patents Act of 1988.

All rights reserved. No part of this publication may be reproduced, stored in or
introduced into a retrieval system, or transmitted in any form or by any means,
electronic, mechanical, photocopying, recording or otherwise, without the prior written
permission of the copyright holder and publisher.

10 9 8 7 6 5 4 3 2 1

A CIP catalogue record for this book is available from the British Library

ISBN   1 904991 18 1

Project editor: Mary Lambert

Photography: Geoff Dann

Printed and bound in Singapore

All rights reserved

ABERDEENSHIRE LIBRARY AND	
INFORMATION SERVICES	
1714481	
HJ	402755
613.704	£14.99
AD	ANF

IMPORTANT HEALTH NOTE

Please be aware that the information contained in this book and the opinions of the author are not
a substitute for medical attention from a qualified health professional. If you are suffering from any
medical complaint, or are worried about any aspect of your health, ask your doctor's advice before
proceeding. The publishers can take no responsibility for any injury or illness resulting from the advice
given, or the poses demonstrated within this volume.

Contents

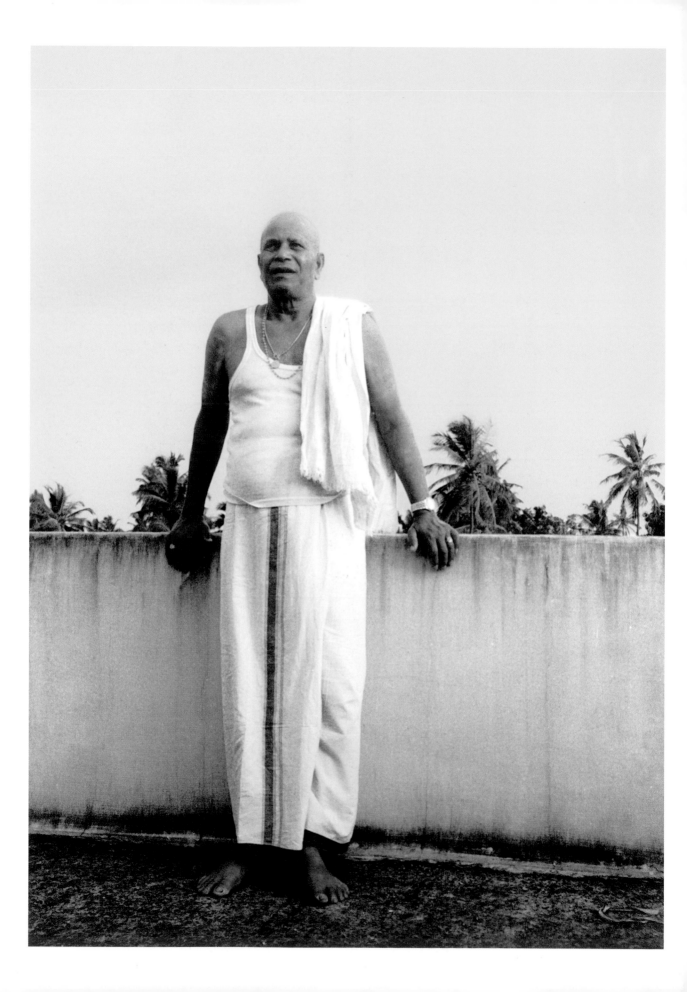

Age can make you either stupid or wise. Stupid means you
still hold on to lots of resentments; you wish you weren't getting old.
Yoga can lift that and bring wisdom and peace.

GURMUKH KAUR KHALSA

Introduction

෧ි

Attaining eternal youthfulness and vitality has been the quest of scientists and philosophers the world over. Plastic surgery, high-impact exercise, and hormone replacement are just a few of the modern answers, sometimes with disastrous side effects. Yoga is a holistic approach that aims at prevention of illness, so that we can age naturally and with grace.

This book is designed to inspire those who wish to defy the conventional model of aging as a process of steady decline, and explore the potential for greater physical and spiritual awareness through the practices of yoga. According to yoga tradition, 50 years of age is the ideal time to develop physically and spiritually, because it is the stage in life when the children have grown, the mind naturally becomes more inward looking, and there is more time to dedicate to the study and practice of yoga. Man has a natural instinct to explore, and yoga is the perfect forum through which to explore the inner workings of the body.

YOGA AND LONGEVITY

Yogis living in India thousands of years ago unlocked the secrets of longevity. Yoga means to yoke or to join, to attach the mind to one object and to penetrate its essential nature. The object that the yogis chose was the human body. They studied intensely the internal activities of the body and mind like digestion, assimilation, expulsion, and breathing, so as to gain ever-greater understanding of its workings. In so doing they became masters of themselves; famous yogis like Krishnamacharya were able to stop their heartbeat at will. Many of the world's most renowned yogis like Indra Devi, B. K. S. Iyengar, Krishnamacharya, and Shree Pattabhi Jois continue practicing and teaching yoga into their 80s, 90s, and 100s, performing complex, mind-bending postures that we would consider impossible past a certain age.

Yoga is a lifestyle, not just a series of exercises. Gerontologists have recently confirmed that biological age can be speeded up or slowed down depending on lifestyle. They have found that adopting a healthy diet, regular exercise and a positive outlook on life can reverse ten years of the traditional signs of aging like high blood pressure, decreased muscle mass, brittle bones, and increased body fat. Slowing down the aging process begins with attention to lifestyle. By improving your diet and with a common-sense approach to maintaining fitness through yoga you can become stronger, increase flexibility, have more energy, and develop a positive outlook.

One of the paradigms of yoga is that "you are as old as your spine." Rounding or curvature of the spine is one of the first signs of aging, which is often accelerated by a sedentary lifestyle. Poor posture affects all the systems of the body, compressing the digestive organs, and restricting breathing. Yoga poses are designed to elongate and maintain the health of the spine and reverse bad postural habits. Also as we age, connective tissue begins to form across the long fibers that make up muscles, causing the muscles to shorten and harden, which affects the arteries. Stretching the muscles daily with yoga asanas breaks up the connective tissue, keeping the muscles soft, young, and supple.

YOGA AS MIND MEDICINE

As well as maintaining the physical body, yoga recognizes and cares for the energetic body (see page 10). According to the principles of yoga, health is experienced when there is an unimpeded flow of prana, or energy, within the body. Asanas combined with breathing and meditation exercises are designed to promote the free flow of energy throughout the body, resulting in greater vitality throughout life; with yoga, we can grow young.

How we think affects the flow of energy in the body. Yoga encourages us to become aware of the stream of life and to embrace and accept change, to focus our awareness on each moment as it arises and then to let it go. The body itself changes from moment to moment until after a seven-year cycle every cell in the body has been renewed. In yoga, it is believed that the more rigid we become in mind, the more rigid in body. Young minds are open and malleable, which is reflected in their natural physical flexibility. The life that flows within the body is like a mountain stream, constantly flowing. The life force is said to have always existed and to be indestructible. The yogi attaches his awareness to the life force, rather than identifying himself with the body and mind that are subjected to old age, sickness, and decay. Yoga helps us face all stages of life calmly yet courageously and encourages us to begin where we are now, in the present.

WHAT THIS BOOK CAN DO FOR YOU

Yoga is a timeless practice that brings body, mind, and spirit into ever-greater harmony. This book is a guide to the physical practices of yoga, including the poses, breathing exercises, and meditation for acquiring radiant health and tranquility. The beauty of yoga is that it can be practiced by anyone, regardless of age or physical ability. Many older students report that they feel in better shape after a few years of practicing yoga than they did in their 40s.

The principal chapters contain simple exercises for warming and limbering all the joints in the body, along with a range of props and exercise variations to make the poses more accessible so that the benefits can be experienced without strain. Asanas for Ailments

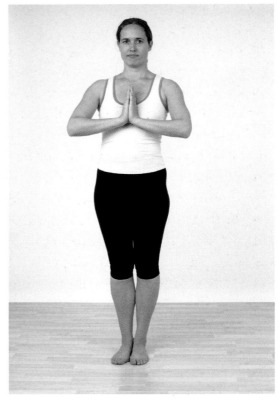

(pages 108–124), presents suitable poses for specific conditions, from improving flexibility in the feet to asanas that help with heart conditions, arthritis, and the menopause. A general workout is included as a guide for daily practice—20 minutes each day will bring you a sense of spontaneity, enjoyment, and well-being.

Yoga is not about self-improvement. It is about self-acceptance.

GURMUKH KAUR KHALSA

Diet

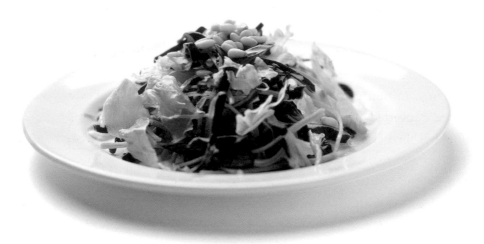

Yoga is more than a set of exercises: it is a complete lifestyle that includes proper eating habits. It is written in the Charaka Samhita that "the life span, complexion, vitality, good health, enthusiasm, plumpness, glow, vital essence, luster, heat and electricity (prana) are derived from the thermogenetic processes in the body," the main one being the "gastric fire." The gastric fire is considered the king of all the metabolic agents in the body, and it is said that proper maintenance of gastric fire is the basis of long life and vitality. There are two important factors in preserving this gastric fire: what we eat, and how we eat.

WHAT WE EAT

Nutrition is now recognized as one of the most important ingredients for prolonged good health. A poor diet high in sugar, animal fat, and sodium, and low in fiber can have disastrous health consequences, and doctors now attribute poor diet as a major contributor to many chronic diseases including heart disease, cancer, and diabetes. Obesity also impacts on the overall health of the body—as many as 40 percent of adults in the US are overweight.

THE YOGI DIET

Yoga's approach to diet is based on common sense. The yogis of old recognized that food contains a vital essence called *prana,* similar to the nutrients in food, which is essential to preserve life. Foods that have the highest level of prana are those that are closest to their natural state and source, for instance, an apple picked straight from a tree. An apple that has been packaged and then has sat around in the supermarket for a while has less vitality, and if it is then taken home and cooked, it loses a little more. In processed food, 90 percent of the nutrients are lost in the processing. That is why we often feel hungry soon after eating a large meal of processed food. The preferred diet of a yogi is one that is rich in natural unmodified foods such as fruit, vegetables, whole grains, nuts, and a little dairy produce. Sprouted grains are particularly high in nutrients as the starch and proteins are converted into nutrients to feed the sprout and then are passed easily into the bloodstream after eating.

Yogis tend to avoid eating meat because they believe in preserving life, and because meat is seen as having little nutritional value (the animal absorbs nutrients from grass and so eating the animal is considered a secondary, rather than primary, source of prana). Yogis also prefer foods that are light and are easily digested, whereas meat takes a long time for the body to break down and process.

However, in yoga it is also recognized that each individual has a unique constitution and requires a different combination of foods for optimum health. Food that is suitable for your body type should leave you feeling light and energetic and bowel movements should be regular and effortless.

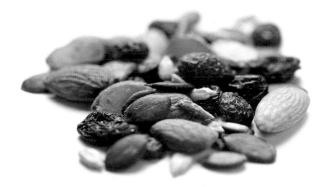

GOOD DIGESTION

Good digestion is recognized by the yoga system as a vital component to staying young and healthy. There is a saying in India that mental clarity comes from a straight spine and a clean colon. Many alternative health professionals also say that most chronic illness begins in the colon. Constipation and other bowel-related illnesses, like irritable bowel syndrome, are among the most prevalent problems in later life. In Indian philosophy, the term for the accumulation of toxins, undigested food, and waste material in the body is *Amma,* which is described as a sticky mucus that blocks the channels of circulation, causes irritable bowel, heaviness, lethargy, bad breath, and painful joints. *Amma* is viewed as a poison that slowly infiltrates the body causing it to break down. Chemically laden food and junk food are difficult for the body to assimilate, so they literally weigh down the body and poison the system.

To keep the digestive system streamlined, yoga advises eating only wholesome foods in smaller portions. When we overload the body with a heavy meal, it requires a lot of vital energy to process and assimilate the food. This takes energy away from being able to think clearly or be physically active, which is why we often feel dull and sleepy after a heavy meal. It is better to eat something light every 2 to 3 hours rather than three heavy meals. Plus as we age, the metabolism slows down and we require less food, although our eating habits do not change. If the system is particularly slow and sluggish, then fasting and internal colon cleansing are both recommended.

WATER

Drink lots of water between meals as this helps to hydrate the system, flushes the kidneys, assists cell function, reduces wrinkles, and helps with elimination of toxins.

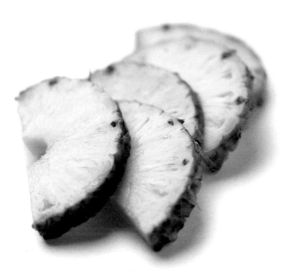

HOW TO EAT

Eating correctly includes how you eat and where you eat. It is important to be calm and relaxed while eating. In our fast-paced society, we are often forced to eat on the run or to grab a bite. Lunch breaks are getting shorter and we often find ourselves eating in front of the computer. When we eat quickly, we do not chew the food well, which is important as the majority of nutrients are absorbed in the mouth, so we are not getting maximum benefit from the food.

Eating a healthy diet does not have to be boring or tasteless. As you feel more energetic, eating the old way will no longer be appealing. Practicing yoga changes the body's cravings, and soon you will find yourself resisting junk food naturally.

Practicing the poses regularly aids the digestion. Many of the yoga asanas are specially designed to put gentle pressure on the colon and intestines, to remove excess gas, and to stimulate the digestive process.

GOOD POSTURE

Posture is important: sitting upright is not just a Victorian hang-up. When we slouch, the "gastric fire" is compressed and breathing, a vital component to digestion, is restricted, making it harder for the body to do the work of digestion and assimilation, causing a build-up of toxins. This is why it is good to take a short slow walk after eating, rather than slouching in front of the TV or going straight to sleep, as the upright posture assists the body's mechanism.

Yoga is not for him who eats too much, nor for one who absolutely abstains from food.
—Bhagavad-Gita VI -16

The Asanas

Asana is the name for the postures of yoga. Yoga asanas include forward bends, backward bends, twists, balancing poses, and inversions. The postures help to tone the muscles and remove the built-up toxins in the body that can cause stiffness in the joints. The poses send oxygen and nutrient-rich blood to nourish every part of the body. The asanas aid digestion, increase circulation, improve concentration, boost the immune system, and generally increase strength and vitality.

FINDING HARMONY

It says in the yoga sutras that whether you are young, old or sick, if you can overcome inertia and laziness, success in the practices of yoga will be attained. Inertia is interpreted as the tendency of the mind to resist change. Humans are creatures of habit, and the older we become the harder it is to make changes and break negative habits. Simply starting yoga can be one of the most difficult obstacles to overcome, especially if you have not exercised in a long time, or are experiencing pain. Many people believe that they have to get fit before they can practice yoga, but the beauty of yoga is that it is available to everyone. The poses can be adapted to a person's needs with the use of numerous props. In yoga, change is embraced as we learn to move with the ebb and flow of life. The poses are difficult initially, because the body is working through a lifetime of habitual patterns of movement. The poses break down old patterns, and awaken new neuromuscular pathways in the brain; breakthrough is experienced as increased freedom and mobility. With regular practice, the poses will become steady and comfortable. Asana literally means steady, comfortable pose.

The body is designed to move in varied and complex ways. One only has to watch the beauty and grace of a ballerina to appreciate the body's potential range of movement. However, with modern life becoming increasingly compartmentalized, our range of motion is being constantly eroded. In the morning we get up from our comfortable mattress, then spend the day sitting at a desk, followed by an evening on a cushioned sofa. Many new injuries are surfacing due to the strain of limited repetitive movements, like carpal tunnel syndrome, which is caused by hours working on a computer.

Yoga practice not only conditions the physical body but it helps to develop our awareness. The presence and focus of mind required for the practice of yoga helps us to become more conscious of the actions that create stiffness in certain muscles and joints, and where we hold stress. Through yoga we can undo any negative postural patterns that contribute to pain and tightness, and return to natural alignment.

Alignment is not a matter of rigidly holding the body in line; rather it is a dynamic process that shifts with each movement. The key to good posture and alignment is that the muscles throughout the body are evenly toned. We tend to use the muscles more on one side of the body than the other, and the ones at the front more than the back. Yoga asanas exercise all the muscles in the body, even minor muscles, keeping the body in a state of dynamic alignment. That is why yoga stretches both sides of the body evenly, and builds muscle tone throughout the body. When the muscles are toned, the joints are fluid, the blood is circulating, the breath is even, and the mind is calm, the body returns to a state of harmony, free from pain.

HOW TO BREATHE

The ideal breath for asana practice is called *ujjai* breathing, whereby you gently contract the glottis to produce a soft snoring sound at the back of the throat while breathing. This action regulates the flow of breath, keeping it steady and even. Inhale slowly and deeply and exhale-completely, emptying the lungs without strain. The breathing should be soft, elongated, and rhythmic like the sound of the ocean. A simultaneous contraction of the abdomen should happen automatically, helping to protect the lower back.

YOGA AND SAFETY

A joint is the point where the end of two bones meet making articulation possible. Each joint is encased in synovial fluid and covered in cartilage, as lubrication is essential for joint mobility. Each joint has a natural range of motion. An inability to move a joint is due to an obstruction,

like a bone deformation, or the muscles that cross the joint being too tight. Stretching the muscles, and gently moving the joints to their full range of motion, as in the warm-up exercises, is the foundation of the yoga practice. Warm-ups prepare the body for the more complicated asanas.

Accidents most often occur due to the overzealousness of the student, who impatiently forces the body into a pose. Yoga has to be practiced with patience, intelligence, and awareness in order to avoid injury. In yoga there is no goal, there is only the journey. Moving in and out of the postures with awareness is just as important as the pose itself.

Always honor pain. A consistent stretching sensation means that the body is working and opening, but a sharp or uncomfortable pain is a signal from the body that something is wrong. If you do not listen to the body's warning signals, an injury may result. It is important to take responsibility for your well-being—even if a teacher tells you to do something but it feels

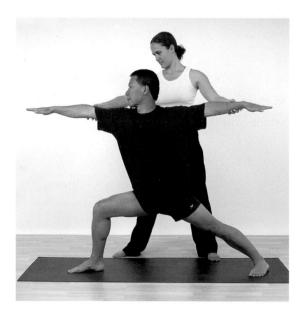

wrong, stop. Yoga is a system of self-knowledge: you have to be truthful and know your own capacity.

CARING FOR THE SPINE

Keeping the spine strong and supple is an essential part of yoga practice. With bad postural alignment the discs get compressed and can rupture or bulge, which is referred to as a slipped disc. The bulging disc can cause pressure on the nerves that results in severe pain, and block the communication between the brain and body, inhibiting movement. In adulthood, all the blood supplied to the spine is derived from movement, without which the discs shrink and lose their elasticity. All the yoga movements accentuate lengthening the spine and increasing the spaces between the discs. Back bends especially are useful for sending fresh blood to the discs and nerves located in the spine.

WHERE AND WHEN

If you are new to yoga or are recovering from illness, I strongly advise that you look for a qualified teacher to learn the basics. To progress, you need to have complete trust and faith in a teacher. It is worth taking your time to try different classes to find a teacher and style with which you feel comfortable.

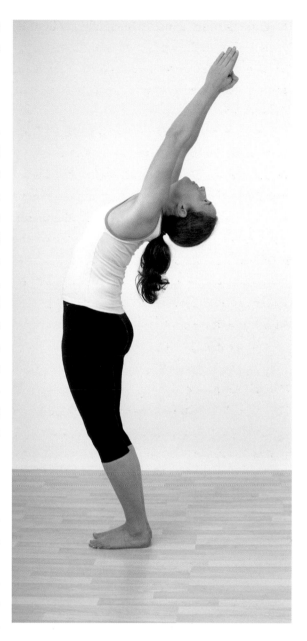

* Yoga can be practiced at any time of day as long as it is 3 hours after food and 1 hour after a caffeinated drink.
* Wear loose comfortable clothing.
* Practice in a warm, draft-free room, and if you are very stiff or suffering from arthritis then a hot bath or a heated room is recommended.

* The room should be clean, quiet, and free from distractions.
* Practice on a soft, slip-free surface. A yoga sticky mat is ideal.
* Anyone suffering from heart problems should not do any poses where the arms are raised over the head.

Thought Patterns

Thoughts are like dynamite. The way we think directly impacts upon the body. In eastern medicine, it is said that all disease has a psychological component. Yoga has the basic principle of mind over matter, and sees the body primarily as a product of consciousness and secondly as a physical object, which is diametrically opposed to the western paradigm that sees the body as a biomechanical organism from which the mind springs.

THE MIND AND BELIEF

The body continually changes as a reflection of the mental state: How we think determines what we become. An image in the mind sends a powerful message through the entire nervous system. The nervous system is a complex network of information. Like a huge telephone exchange, it consists of the central nervous system, the brain and spinal cord, the somatic nervous system, which is in contact with the outside world, and autonomic nervous system that controls internal mechanisms like heart rate, or blood pressure. The thoughts running through the nervous system trigger hormones to be released into the blood which impact our physical body and appearance. When we are angry our face becomes red, the brow tenses up and the blood pressure rises. Recent scientific research has verified the link between the mind and the body; findings show that someone suffering from depression is four times more likely to develop disease. Depression or stress creates havoc with the immune system, sending a tidal wave of destructive hormones into the blood stream, which saps the life force. No thought or emotion is without electrochemical activity, which sends messages through which the body. The body is a field of energy in continual flux that is renewing itself every second.

Each time that someone asked Jesus to perform a miracle, Jesus would first ask the onlooker, "Do you believe?" Belief forms the bedrock in our minds of how and when things can happen. Believing yourself old, you will become old. In cultures that have a positive

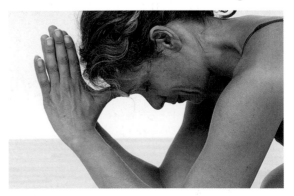

image of aging, a person is thought to become wiser with age and more able to lead the community, chronic age-related illnesses, like heart attacks and arthritis, are relatively nonexistent. Aging is fluid and changeable, which continually baffles scientists, as there is no consistent pattern. Each person experiences aging differently, depending on their response to the external world, which in turn influences their mental state.

Negative thoughts produce negative results. The way we think affects the body's nerves, glands, and energy channels. Negative thoughts choke and stifle the flow of energy through the channels; positive feelings like joy or love cause the energy channels to open, which is why we feel a rush of energy and are more buoyant and energetic when in love. Positive thinking and affirmations are an integral part of yoga practice, as a way to redirect mental energy and trigger a constructive chemical response in the body. Eric Shiffman, *Yoga: The Spirit of Practice and Moving Into Stillness,* says "When you catch yourself imagining an undesirable future like, 'my health will just get worse,' be aware you are thinking this, pause, cancel the thought, and take a moment to feel the creative life force which is what you are. Don't believe the negative projections; instead feel the energy that constitutes you. This way you leave a space for the miraculous to occur."

In my experience I find that many people who enter a yoga class have already decided what they can and cannot do before they even start a pose. But I cannot stress enough the importance of an open mind. When the mind is

---

According to yoga scripture, the body is made of five layers, like an onion, each level more subtle than the previous one:

1. *Annamaya Kosha:* the physical body

The physical body is considered to be the aspect of ourselves with which we most identify.

2. *Pranamaya Kosha:* the energy body

The energy body is made up of a network of 72,000 energy channels, or *nadis,* that span our entire bodies, the channels radiating from certain energy centers called *chakras,* meaning wheels. The energy that moves through the channels is called *prana,* or life force; it is like a wind that moves and animates the physical body.

3. *Manomaya Kosha:* the mind body

Our thought patterns determine how energy flows through the body. Thoughts are said to be like a subtle vibration that stirs the inner winds or energy body that then incites the body into action.

4. *Vijnanamaya Kosha:* awareness

Awareness is a field of pure perception, which can be experienced during deep meditation as a silent witness to our thoughts and reactions.

5. *Anandamaya Kosha:* the field of limitless potential The energy moves from the center outward just like the concentric ripples on the surface of a pond from the field of potential out to the physical body.

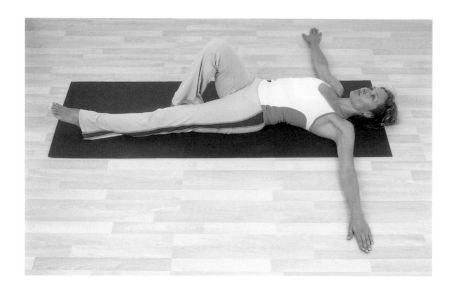

present in each moment free of expectation, then miracles can happen and the body can move in new and unfamiliar ways.

The purpose of yoga is to harness the tremendous energy of the mind. The poses and the breathing techniques deliberately open and redirect the flow of energy that in turn calms the mind and changes habitual ways of thinking. When the energies of the mind are harnessed through meditation they can be directed toward accomplishing any goal. The complicated movements of yoga are the first step in training the mind, through developing concentration. Concentration is necessary to carry out the complicated movements, and to hold the poses. Even thinking about performing an exercise has

benefits: when you think about a certain area of the body electrical impulses increase in that area. For someone in too much pain to do the physical asana, just visualizing the poses has a positive effect and promotes healing. The medical community, with startling results, has studied the effects of biofeedback. Using a biofeedback machine, doctors have shown that it is possible to control and change such autonomic body functions as blood pressure, heart rate, circulation, digestion, and perspiration. A positive, kind attitude toward your body is important. Even if it is causing you pain and you are frustrated, sending positive thoughts helps to change negative patterns and promote healing.

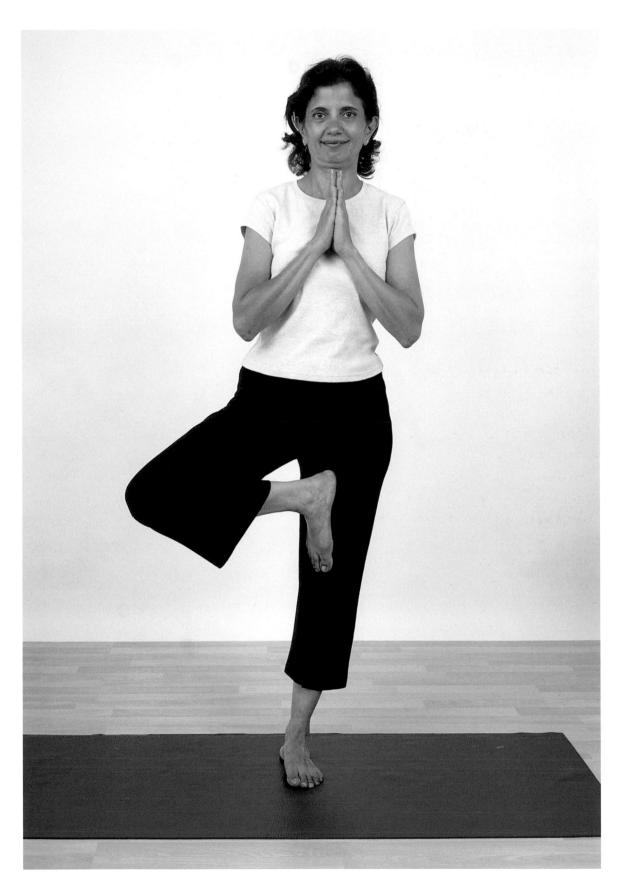

Yoga and the Breath

According to the wisdom of yoga, breathing is much more than the intake of oxygen. Air is believed to contain a subtle energy called *prana*. Prana is the energy, or life force, that animates our physical world. The Chinese refer to it as *chi*. It is said that when prana is not flowing in the body, old age and sickness are the result. Prana is increased not only through the breath but is also absorbed from food, especially fresh produce, and from sunlight and physical exercise, particularly yoga asanas. Conservation of prana increases health and vitality. You look and feel better: the mind becomes clear and is less disturbed by the ups and downs of life.

PRANAYAMA

The method of rhythmically controlling the breath is called *pranayama,* which literally means "expansion of the life force." Yogis discovered that by manipulating the breath they could control prana. Advanced breath control is not taught until a person has mastered the physical poses. However, the following breathing exercises are preparatory exercises that can be practiced at any level and are an easy starting point for any one in severe pain or has a chronic disease and is unable to do the physical movements of yoga. They are generally practiced after the asanas, at the end of a yoga workout, followed by meditation (see page 87).

Always breathe through the nose, as the nose naturally filters out dust and particles from the air and also warms the air to the perfect temperature for assimilation by the lungs. If you find that one nostril is blocked, release it by making a fist and placing it under the opposite armpit from the blocked nostril. Apply pressure with the upper arm and hold for a few minutes.

Never strain when practicing breathing exercises. They are designed to deepen relaxation, so if you feel agitated and tense then stop and rest. Always practice on an empty stomach. Sit upright in a chair; or crosslegged on a cushion; lean your back against a wall for added support if you need to.

CLEANSING PRANAYAMA

The following two breaths are purifying or cleansing techniques, and are used to remove toxins from the body.

Shining Skull Breath *Kapalabhati*

This rapid diaphragmatic breathing removes carbon dioxide and impurities from the body and clears the sinuses and lungs.

Quickly contract the abdomen to exhale. Relax the abdomen and air will automatically be drawn into the lungs. Follow these two movements in quick succession, so it sounds like a train chugging along. Do 3 to 5 rounds with 20 to 30 contractions per round. Release and take a deep breath, then an extended exhalation, and return to normal breathing. If you feel dizzy, stop or slow down the contractions.

Lion Breath *Simhaasana*

Lion breath is an easy cleansing exercise that serves a dual purpose of helping to remove stale oxygen from the lungs and exerting pressure on the abdomen to eliminate waste.

1. Sit in a chair or kneel on the floor. Open the knees and place the hands on the floor with fingertips pointing toward the body. Lean forward, taking the weight onto the hands. Inhale gradually and slowly through the nose.

2. Exhale from the back of the throat through an open mouth, while stretching the tongue out toward the chin. At the end of the exhalation, suck the belly in and up to form a hollow beneath the ribcage. Hold for a moment, and then gradually breathe in through the nose and rest. Repeat 3 to 5 times.

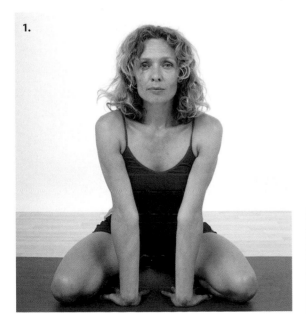

1.

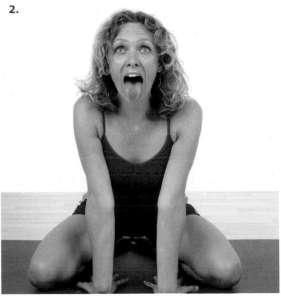

2.

CALMING PRANAYAMA

Rhythmic Breathing

Rhythmic breathing reflects the way that babies breathe and the breathing pattern during deep, relaxed sleep. This breathing technique uses the diaphragm and minimizes the action of the rib cage. The technique activates the lower lobes of the lung while the action of the diaphragm also massages the liver and stomach and aids digestion.

This is a very simple, calming breath. It is a useful exercise while lying in bed to aid sleep.

Place one or both hands on the belly. As you inhale, gently relax the belly until you feel the belly pushing against your hands. On the exhalation, draw the belly back toward the spine. This breath can be practiced for as long as it is comfortable.

Full Yogic Breath *Deergha Swaasam*

Full yogic breath is an extension of rhythmic breathing, whereby the inhalation and exhalation is lengthened with the use of the rib cage. Indra Devi, the first lady of yoga, who lived and practiced yoga daily until aged 102, recommended 60 deep breaths a day. It takes time to build up the intercostal muscles and the lungs, so take it slowly and build up over time and start with a few rounds.

Breathing deeply comprises a three-step process.

1. Inhale by expanding the abdomen, drawing air to the lower lung.

2. Expand the rib cage out to the sides taking air into the middle of the lung.

3. Lift the collarbones, bringing air to the top of the lung. Exhale in reverse order, releasing the breath from the upper lung, middle lung, and then drawing in the belly. Make both the inhalation and exhalation one continuous flow. Repeat the breath 3 to 5 times, end on an exhalation, then return to normal breathing.

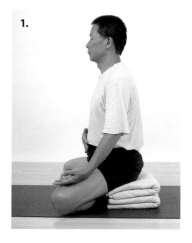
1.

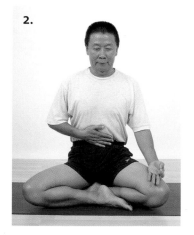
2.

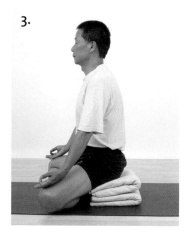
3.

Nerve Purification Breath *Nadi Suddhi*

In this technique, the breath is through alternate nostrils, which is a very powerful method of calming and relaxing the nervous system. When we breathe through the right nostril, which is called surya, the sun channel, it activates the left side of the brain, which governs the sympathetic nervous system. When we breathe through the left nostril, chandra, the moon channel, the right side of the brain is activated. By breathing through alternate nostrils, the nervous system is brought into harmony and balance.

1. Sit on the floor in a comfortable meditation posture with the spine erect. Bend the right arm and take the right hand into *Vishnu mudra* by closing the forefingers and index fingers. Relax the face.

Close the right nostril with the thumb. Completely exhale all the air from the lungs through the left nostril without strain, then slowly and deeply inhale through the same nostril to the count of four. Expand the stomach and chest to pull in more air, without strain.

2. Next close the left nostril with the ring finger and release the right nostril. Very slowly exhale making the exhalation longer than the inhalation. With practice, the exhalation should be twice the length of the inhalation, but do not rush it. Then inhale through the same nostril, close the right nostril and open the left nostril and repeat the cycle. Perform at least ten rounds. Release, and return to normal breathing.

Vishnu Mudra

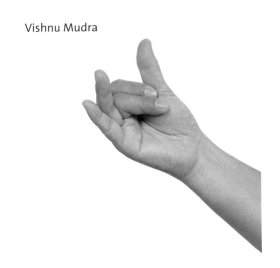

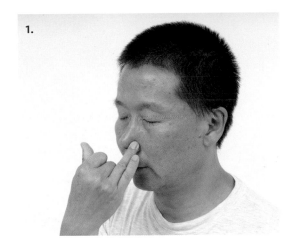

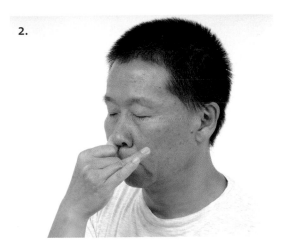

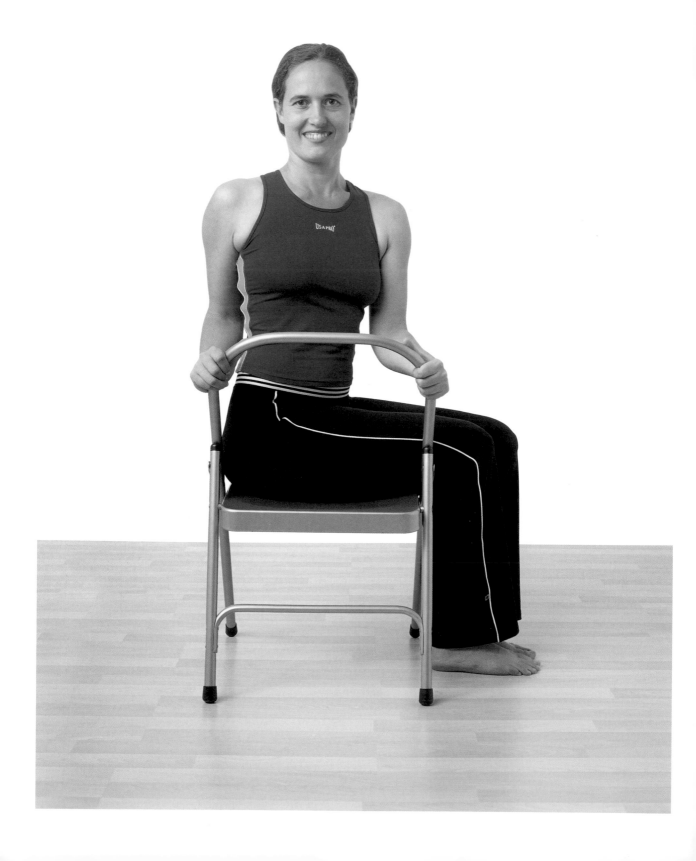

CHAPTER 1

Working with Props

The use of props was pioneered by the great Indian yogi B. K. S. Iyengar, and has since been adopted by many schools of yoga. A prop can be any object as long as it is sturdy, will support the required weight, and helps you to practice a pose safely. Props are especially useful for beginners, or anyone with injuries, because they help you navigate around old injuries, allowing the body to experience a pose in an open, more relaxed way. Using a supportive prop also gives the nervous system time to become accustomed to a pose, so that later it may be practiced more easily. Many experienced yoga practitioners also enjoy using props as part of restorative practice, which involves using gentler versions of complete poses. Props allow you to hold the poses for much longer, without undue strain.

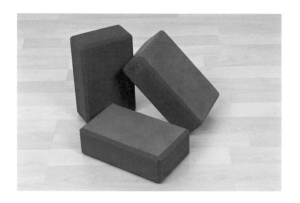

Blocks

Yoga blocks are made of wood or lightweight foam. Blocks can be used in myriad ways and are especially useful for people with less flexibility, allowing them to practice the poses without strain.

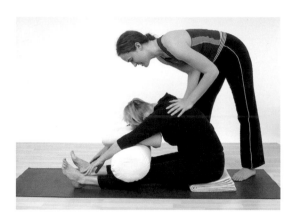

Bolster

A bolster is a long firm cushion that is a perfect prop for a range of restorative poses. Restorative poses are gentle, relaxing adaptations of complete poses that are useful when a person is low in energy, experiencing a life change such as menopause, or if recovering from illness or injury.

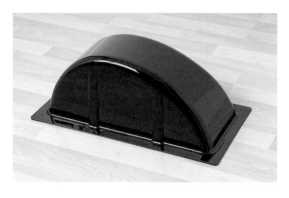

Back arch

A back arch is a great way to gently flex and elongate the spine without fear of injury. Lying over an arch provides the perfect counter-stretch after a day working at a desk. The back arch gently arcs over into a deeper curve.

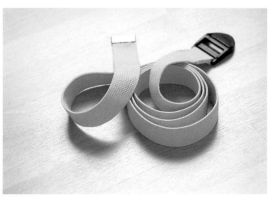

Belt

A belt is useful for new practitioners, helping users to extend their reach and easily access poses like forward bends, or other poses in which the hands need to reach the feet or clasp together behind the back.

Blanket

A blanket is a great basic prop—you can easily fold it to allow for additional lift and height in forward bends and shoulder stands, as well as using it as a cover to keep the body warm during relaxation.

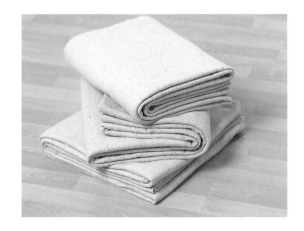

Chair

A chair is one of the most versatile props, especially for those who are stiff and new to yoga and have difficulty sitting on the floor, or getting down to or up from the floor. A chair helps maintain balance for older practitioners who fear falling; it also promotes the necessary strength so that you become less dependent upon it. A regular metal fold-up chair is best. Choose one that is robust with a large enough gap between the seat and the back rest to allow the legs to slide easily through the back.

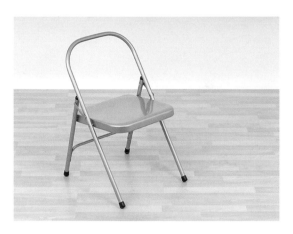

Wall

A section of bare wall is perhaps the simplest of props, and the perfect teacher of alignment. Standing in *tadasana,* with the back to the wall, helps us discover how far we have strayed from an upright position. A wall is a great support for inversions, providing a useful way to ease into shoulder stand, and a support for both handstand and headstand.

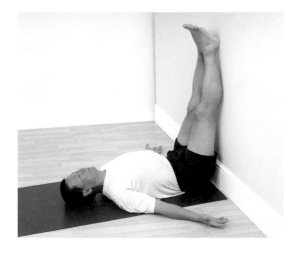

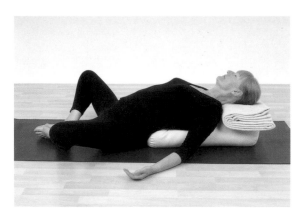

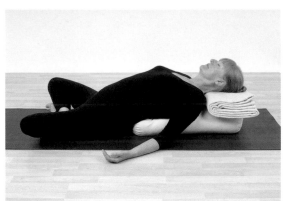

Cobbler pose with a bolster
Supta Baddha Konasana

Sit in *dandasana* (see page 79). Place a bolster behind you, lengthwise, and have ready a folded blanket by your mat. Bend the knees and draw the soles of your feet together, close to the groin. Relax the knees out to the sides; inhale. Exhale, lie back on the bolster so that the ribs are supported and the spine is on the center of the bolster. Place the blanket under the head to relieve neck tension. Tuck the chin in slightly, to extend the back of the neck, and relax the face. Relax the arms out to the sides, palms up, and the shoulders relaxed down. To deepen relaxation, inhale slowly and deeply and exhale slowly, emptying the lungs without strain. Breathing should be soft, elongated and rhythmic like the sound of the ocean. Hold for 5 to 10 minutes.

BENEFITS   Using a bolster in *supta virasana* or *baddha konasana* can help during menopause as they release the pelvis and regulate hormone production; these poses also aid digestion.

✳ TIP   If the legs are uncomfortable in *baddha konasana*, then simply cross the feet at the ankles to form *sukhasana*.

Hero pose with a bolster *Supta Virasana*

Kneel on the mat. Place a bolster on the mat behind you so that the top of the bolster touches the base of the ribs. Lift up onto the knees and separate the feet. Gently sit back and ease the buttocks down between the feet. If you experience strain in the knees, place a folded blanket under the buttocks or widen the knees. Gently lower down onto the bolster so that the spine is on the center of the bolster. Place a folded blanket under the head for additional support. Breathe deeply and rhythmically. Hold the pose for 5 to 10 minutes.

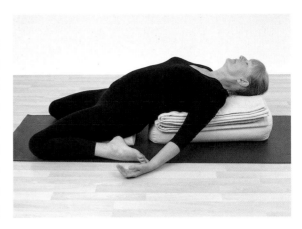

Downward dog with a bolster

Adho Mukha Svanasana

Place a bolster on the mat lengthwise. Come onto all fours with hands palms down on either side of the bolster, close to the far end. Tuck the toes under, inhale, and push up into downward dog. Relax the head and shoulders and place the forehead on the bolster. Breathe steadily; hold for 5 to 10 minutes. Exhale to come down.

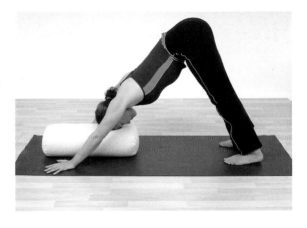

✳ **TIP** If you experience strain in the knees when lowering down onto the bolster, raise the height of the bolster using folded blankets.

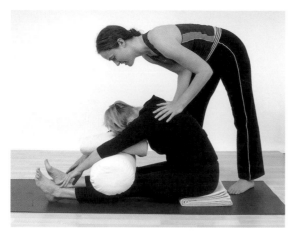

Forward bend with a bolster

Paschimottanasana

Sit in *dandasana* (see page 79). Place a bolster across the legs. Inhale, lift up and elongate the spine. Exhale and bend forward, placing the forehead on the top of the bolster. Relax the arms over the bolster to form a gentle forward bend. Breathe steadily and easily. Hold for 5 to 10 minutes.

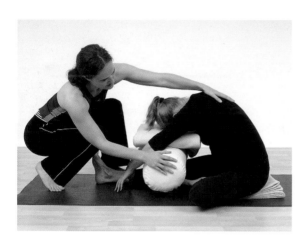

Head-to-knee pose with a bolster

Janu Sirsasana

Sit in *dandasana* (see page 79). Bend the left leg and place the sole of the left foot along the inside of the right thigh. Place a bolster across the extended left leg. Inhale, lift up and lengthen the spine. Exhale and bend forward over the extended leg. Place the forehead on top of the bolster. Relax the arms forward over the bolster. Breathe steadily and evenly. Hold for 5 to 10 minutes, then repeat on the opposite side.

BENEFITS Relaxing the head forward rests the heart and sends a supply of oxygen-rich blood to the brain.

✳ **TIP** If it is not possible to place the forehead easily on the bolster, place a folded blanket on top of the bolster for added height.

Side twist with a chair *Bharadvajasana*

Sit sideways on the chair, with the back of the chair in the direction of the twist. Place the ankles directly under the knees with the feet and knees together. Inhale, sit up, lift the chest and elongate the spine. Exhale and turn to the right. Hold the chair back with both hands, and use the back of the chair to pull deeper into the twist. Twist from the base of the spine, then the navel and the chest. Look over the right shoulder and hold for 8 breaths. Repeat on the opposite side.

BENEFITS   Both the side twist and the forward bend with a chair are invaluable poses for anyone suffering from back stiffness.

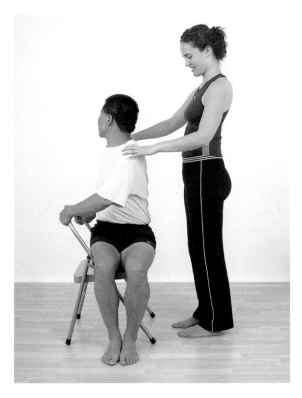

Forward bend with a chair *Uttanasana*

Sit on a chair so that the buttocks are close to the back of the chair seat. Place the feet on the outsides of the front chair legs, so that the soles of the feet are flat on the floor. Inhale and elongate the spine, then exhale and fold forward between the knees and relax the upper body down over the front of the chair. Relax the neck and shoulders. Now hold the pose for a few minutes, breathing evenly. Slowly curl up, one vertebra at a time.

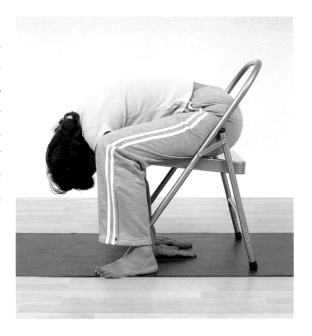

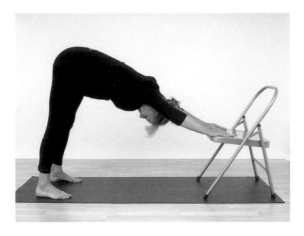

Downward dog with a chair
Adho Mukha Svanasana

Place a chair at one end of the yoga mat with the seat facing toward you. Inhale, then exhale as you bend forward, placing the heels of both hands so that they rest at the front edge of the chair. Walk the feet backward about 3 to 4 feet (1 to 1.2 m) from the chair. Now press away from the front of the chair with both hands, and lift the pelvis high. Flatten the back and look down between the arms. Hold the pose for 20 to 30 seconds, breathing evenly, then exhale as you release and come down.

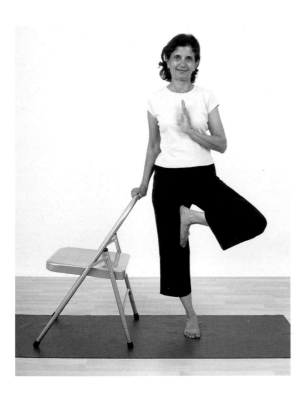

Tree pose with a chair *Vrksasana*

Place a chair on the mat and stand next to it with the back of the chair toward you. Come into tree pose using the back of the chair for support, slowly lifting and bending the left leg up and out to the side then resting the sole of the foot on the right thigh. Hold for 8 breaths then repeat on the opposite side.

✳ **TIP** This variation further flexes the hip joints. Holding the back of the chair for support, slowly lift and bend the right leg. Take hold of the right foot, placing it as high up the left thigh as is comfortable, with the sole facing up. Hold for 8 breaths.

Plow pose with a chair *Halasana*

1. Place a folded blanket on the mat and chair seat; place the chair next to the blanket, so the front legs touch the edge of the blanket. Lie on the blanket with the shoulders parallel to its edge and the head underneath the chair seat. Place the hands alongside the hips, with the palms face down. Inhale, and on an exhalation bend the knees in toward the chest and swing the legs up over the head. Support the back with both hands.

2. Extend the feet through the back of the chair and place the tops of the thighs on the seat of the chair. Once the legs are supported release the hands and extend the arms on the floor away from the feet.

3. Interlock the hands and stretch the arms away to come higher onto the shoulders. Relax the face. Breathe steadily and hold for 1 to 3 minutes.

4. To release, slowly roll out, supporting the buttocks with the hands. Relax, with the knees toward the chest.

1.

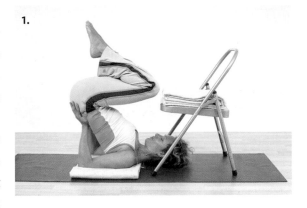

2.

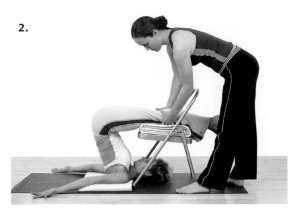

3.

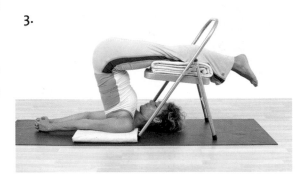

4.

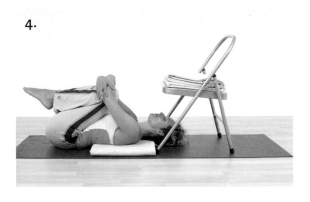

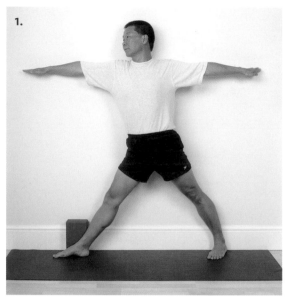

1.

Triangle pose with a block *Trikonasana*
Blocks can act as useful hand rests in most standing poses. Place the block on or near the mat, within easy reach.

1. Stand in *tadasana* (see page 60). If you need to, rest the back against a wall for additional support. Step the feet 3 to 4 feet (1 to 1.2 m) apart. Rotate the right foot and leg out toward the end of the mat and turn the left foot into a 45-degree angle. Keep the pelvis facing forward. Place the block on the outside of the right ankle. Inhale, lift the arms to shoulder height, and extend out to the fingertips.

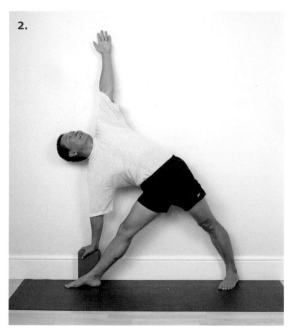

2.

2. Exhale and lean to the right, keeping the chest and pelvis facing forward. Place the right hand on the top of the block. Extend the left arm up, so that the arms form a vertical line. Turn the head to look up toward the left hand. Hold for 8 breaths. Repeat on the opposite side.

BENEFITS Triangle poses remove stiffness in the legs and hips, stretching the intercostal muscles of the ribs, which helps to improve breathing capacity.

Bridge pose with a block

Setu Bandhasana

Bend the legs, stretch the arms toward the feet, and hold the ankles. Tuck the tailbone under; inhale. Exhale, pushing into the heels and lifting the pelvis. Roll onto the shouldertops and lift the chest. Place a horizontal block underneath the sacrum. With the arms relaxed, tuck the chin to gently stretch through the neck. Hold for 8 breaths. Exhale, lift the pelvis (see right), remove the block. Release, relaxing one vertebra at a time.

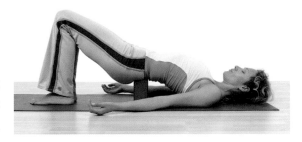

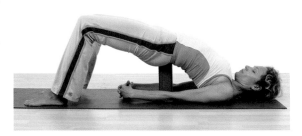

✳ **TIP** If you are comfortable with the block placed horizontally, and depending on the flexibility of your spine, you can place the block vertically. Clasp the hands and push down with the arms and sides of the hands to raise the pelvis higher, then ask a partner to position the block vertically.

Cobbler pose with blocks

Baddha Konasana

Sit in *dandasana* (see page 79) with the legs outstretched. Bend both knees and bring the feet in toward you as close to the groin as possible. Touch the soles of the feet together, and drop the knees to the sides. Place a block underneath each knee for support. Hold the feet and keep the spine straight and lifted. Hold the pose for 20 to 30 seconds or longer, breathing evenly.

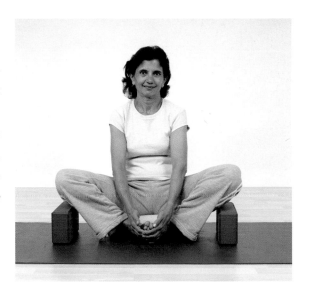

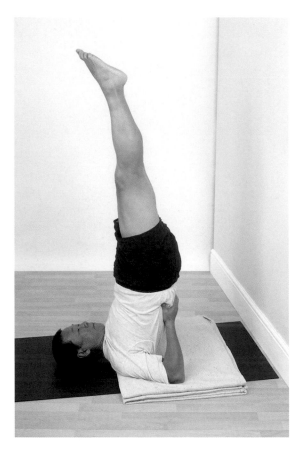

Shoulder stand with a blanket
Salamba Sarvangasana

Fold a blanket so that it is wide enough for the shoulders. Make sure that the edge of the blanket the shoulders are against is neatly folded and straight. Lie on the blanket so that the tops of the shoulders are in line with the edge of the folded blanket.

Tuck the chin in slightly and lengthen through the back of the neck. Place the arms alongside the body with the palms down. Exhale and bend the knees. Push into the palms and begin to raise the legs over the head. Bend the arms and place the hands in the middle of the back on either side of the spine to support the back, without widening the elbows.

Bring the torso to a vertical position moving the chest toward the chin. Straighten the legs to a vertical position, in line with the torso. Aim for a straight line between the shoulders, hips, and ankles. Tuck the tailbone under and lengthen along the spine. Remember to relax the muscles in the face. Stay breathing quietly for at least one minute. Come down carefully by placing the palms of the hands down flat on the floor and rolling down slowly, one vertebra at a time.

✳ **TIP** Most people are stiff in the lower back and hips, which means that when they sit directly on the mat, the base of the spine tends to bow outward.

To compensate for the tightness, sit up on a folded blanket so that the hips are higher than the knees, in order to protect the lower back during forward bends like *paschimottonasana* and *janu sirsasana* (see pages 81, 82).

Half-lotus *Ardha Padmaasana*

Sit on a folded blanket or block to raise the hips and ease the lower back. Bend the left leg and place the left foot close to the groin with the sole of the foot facing up. Bend the right leg and, carefully taking hold of the ankle, lift the right foot up over the left leg and onto the top of the left thigh with the sole of the right foot facing up. Lift the chest, lengthen the spine, and place the hands on top of the knees. Hold for 20 to 30 seconds. Release the legs and repeat on the opposite side.

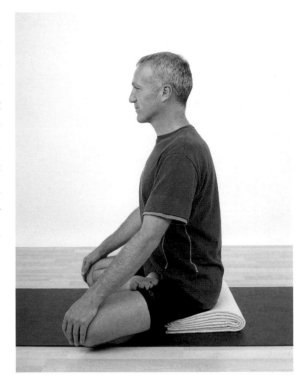

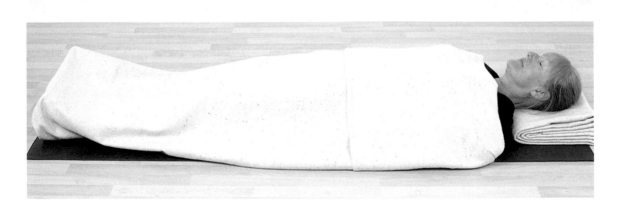

Savasana with a blanket *Savasana*

After practicing yoga asanas it is highly recommended that you rest for ten minutes in *savasana*. This pose, in which you lie comfortably on your back, gives the body time to deeply relax and absorb the full benefits of the practice. Also, because the body's temperature rises during the practice and the muscles become warm, it is important not to lose heat too quickly from the body as this causes shock to the system. Unless it is a really hot day, always wrap up for *savasana*—put on socks and a cardigan, if you have one with you, and cover yourself with a blanket—to retain heat, as the body temperature drops dramatically during relaxation.

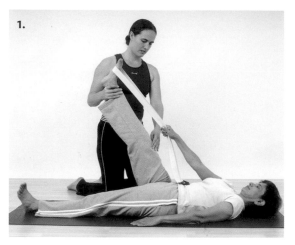

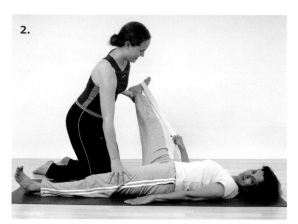

Lying thumb-to-foot pose with a belt

Supta Padangusthasana

1. Lie flat on the back with legs and feet together. Bend the right leg in toward the chest and place a belt around the ball of the right foot.

2. Take hold of both ends of the belt with the right hand. Straighten the right leg up, stretching into the heel of the right foot. Keep the right shoulder down, the hips level, and the left leg strong by pushing into the ground with the left thigh. Keep the left arm alongside the body with the palm down. Inhale. Exhale and extend the right leg out to the right side as far as is comfortable. Turn the head to look over the left shoulder. Hold for 8 breaths. Repeat on the opposite side.

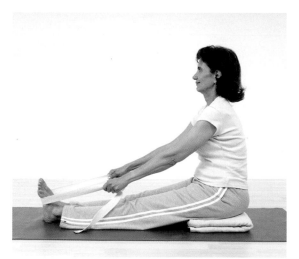

Seated forward with a belt

Paschimottanasana

Sit in *dandasana* (see page 79). Bend the knees and place a belt around the balls of both feet, then straighten the legs. Inhale; lift the chest and elongate the spine. Exhale. Bend forward with a flat back and grasp the belt as close to the feet as possible. Take the elbows to the sides and the head toward the knees. Relax the back of the neck and shoulders. Keep the thighs pressed into the floor. Hold for 8 breaths. Inhale and come up.

Tree pose with a belt *Vrksasana*

Stand in *tadasana* (see page 60) and spread the toes. Begin to take the body weight into the left leg. Bend the right leg and place a belt around the right ankle so that the belt wraps around the thigh. Use the belt to lift the foot as high as possible and place the sole of the foot on the inside of the left leg. Keep hold of the belt with the right hand. Hold for 8 breaths, breathing steadily and evenly. Repeat on the opposite side.

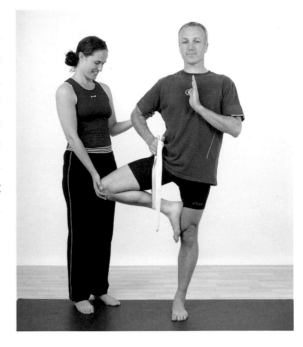

✳ **TIP** An alternative to wrapping the belt around the ankle and thigh is to loop one end of the belt. Slip the loop over the right foot and onto the right ankle. Gently use the other end of the belt to lift the right leg up and place the sole of the right foot as far as possible on the inside of the left leg.

Cow-face pose with a belt

Gomukhasana

Sit with the legs out straight. Bend the left leg so the knee is in line with the center of the body. Place the heel on the floor by the right hip. Bend the right leg over the left, so that the heel is in line with the left hip.

Holding a belt in the right hand, raise the right arm. Bend the right elbow and reach the right hand behind the back of the neck. Bend the left arm behind the back at waist level and grasp the belt. Work the left hand closer to the right hand using the belt. Keep the head and neck straight. Hold for 8 breaths, breathing evenly. Repeat on the opposite side.

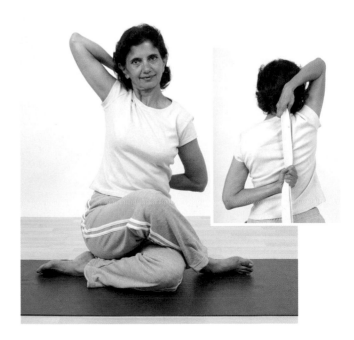

1.

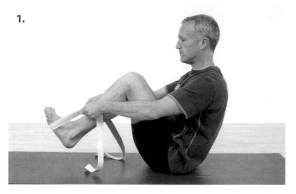

2.

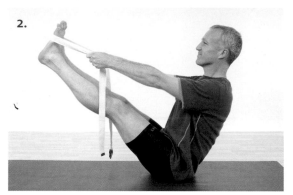

1.

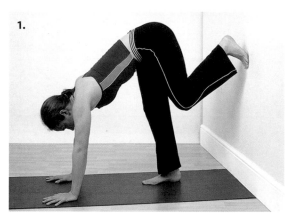

2.

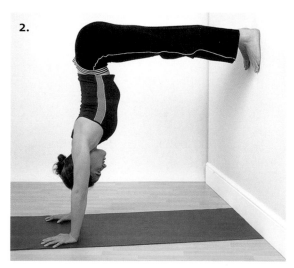

Boat pose *Navasana*

1. Sit with your legs outstretched in front. Bend the knees and place a belt around the balls of the feet. Hold the belt in both hands and slowly lean back until you are balancing on your buttocks.

2. When you are balanced, inhale then exhale as you slowly straighten the knees and extend the legs. Keep hold of the belt. Draw in the belly and lift the chest. Hold for 8 breaths, breathing evenly in the pose.

Half-handstand with a wall
Ardha Vrksasana

1. Practice the half-handstand using a wall for support as a way to build up the strength and confidence necessary for the full handstand. Stand with your back to the wall. Squat down and place the hands on the mat about 3 to 4 feet (1 to 1.2 m) from the wall. Raise the hips. Bend the left knee and place the sole of the left foot on the wall at hip height.

2. Shift the body weight into the hands. Press the left foot into the wall and lift the right foot up in line with the left foot. Press into both feet and straighten the legs to form a right angle between the legs and the torso. Hold for 10 to 20 seconds and carefully come down one foot at a time. Return to a squatting position for a few moments before standing.

Handstand with a wall
Adho Mukha Vrksasana

1. Squat down. Place the hands, palms down and shoulder-width apart, on the floor in front of you, 6 inches (15 cm) from the wall.

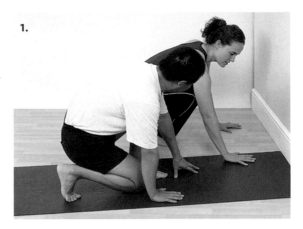

2. Raise the hips, straighten the arms, and begin to bring the body weight into the hands. Inhale and on an exhale, kick the right leg up toward the wall followed by the left. Push up from the palms, straighten the elbows, and lift the shoulders and chest. Tuck the tailbone in to reduce the arch in the back. Bring the feet together, make the legs strong, and extend the heels upward. Breathe 8 or more times and come down by dropping one leg toward the floor. Return to a squatting position for a few minutes before standing.

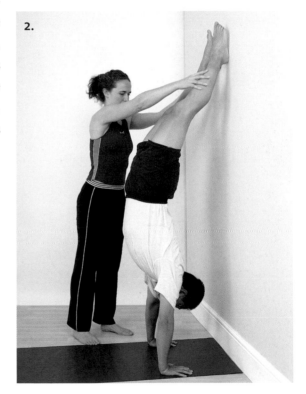

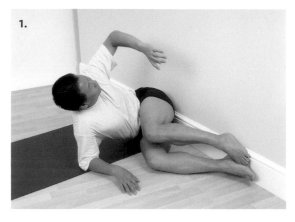

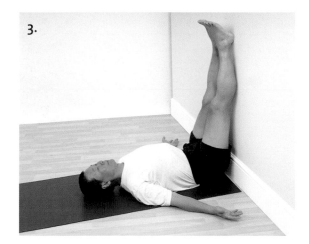

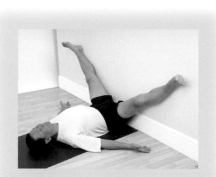

Legs up the wall *Viparita Karani*

1. Sit sideways and shift the buttocks close to the wall, with the left hip pointing up.

2. Once the buttocks are in place, release the side of the torso to the floor, roll over onto the back, and raise the legs up the wall.

3. Straighten through the backs of the legs, so that the backs are touching the wall. Tuck the chin in slightly and lengthen through the back of the neck. Flex the feet and extend through the backs of the legs. Relax the arms alongside the body. Hold for 10 to 15 minutes.

✳ **TIP** To stretch the inside of the legs and to create flexibility in the hips, practice the pose with the legs apart.

Half-moon pose *Ardha Chandrasana*

1. Stand with your back against a wall with the feet 3 to 4 feet (1 to 1.2 m) apart. Turn the right leg and foot out toward the end of the mat and turn the back foot in slightly. Extend the arms out to the sides. Inhale, and on an exhalation bend the right leg and place the fingertips of the right hand on the floor or on a block about 1.5 feet (just over a meter) in front of the right foot. Draw the back foot in slightly. At the same time, straighten the right leg and lift the left leg up until it is parallel with the floor.

2. Extend the left arm so that both arms form a straight line against the wall. Keep rotating the chest and lifting the left hip so that the body is on one plane. Stretch into the heel of the left leg. Turn the head to look up toward the left thumb. Maintain the weight in the standing leg, not the arm. Breathe steadily for 8 breaths. Repeat the pose on the other side.

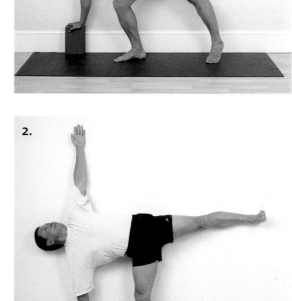

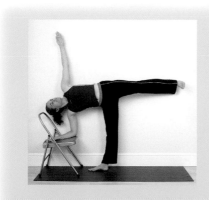

✳ **TIP** To make the pose even more accessible, practice the pose using a chair for additional height and support.

Opening the upper chest and neck

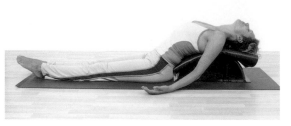

Sit in *dandasana* (see page 79) with your bottom at the base of the arch. Gently lower yourself backward onto the arch. Now relax the head and neck, soften the shoulders and open the chest. Focus on opening up the heart center, or chakra, in the chest. Breathe steadily and evenly for 10 minutes.

Opening the thorax, spine, and side ribs

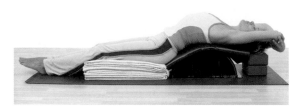

Place 3 or 4 folded blankets at the base of the back arch and two blocks at the back of the arch. Sit in *dandasana* (see page 79) at the base of the arch. Gently lower yourself backward over the back arch, allowing the back of the head to be supported by the blocks. Extend the arms over the head and take hold of opposite elbows. Enjoy the stretch, breathing easily for 5 to 10 minutes.

Opening the lower back and pelvis

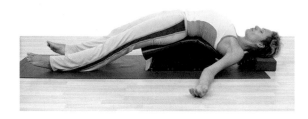

Sit part way up the back arch, then gently lower yourself backward over the arch. Place a block under the back of the head for additional support. Extend the legs away. Allow the arms to fall naturally to the sides with the palms facing up. Relax for 10 to 15 minutes.

✳ **TIP** Depending upon where you lie on the arch (see also page 26) the back arch will stretch a different part of the back. Made from molded plastic, a back arch can feel hard, slippery, and generally uncomfortable without padding, so it is advisable to place it on top of a sticky mat and then fold a second sticky mat over the arch for additional support. Detailed here are four variations using the back arch. Some of the exercises use blocks and blankets (see pages 26, 27) which (as with all poses) you should place within easy reach of your mat before you begin.

Half-shoulder stand with a back arch

Sit on the top of the back arch. Gently lower yourself back over the arch until the shoulders are on the mat. Tuck the chin in and extend through the back of the neck. Lift the legs up into a vertical position, one leg at a time. Place the hands on the floor with palms facing down-ward, alongside the arch. Relax for 5 minutes, breathing evenly.

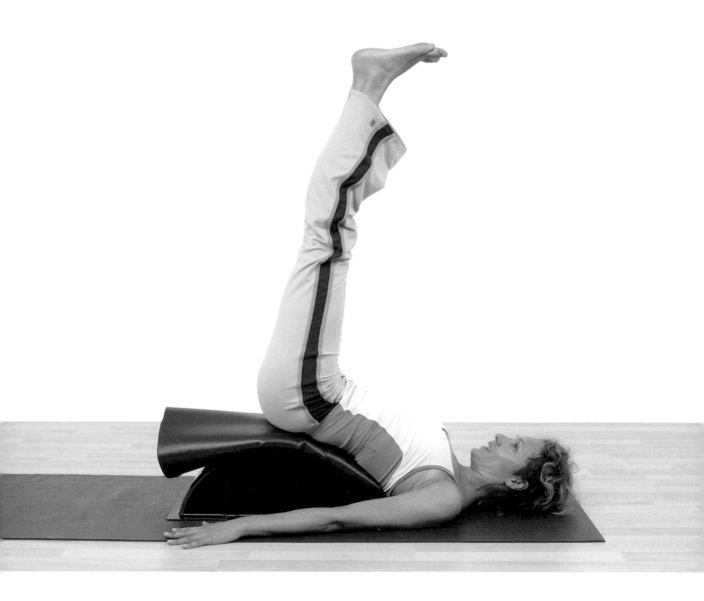

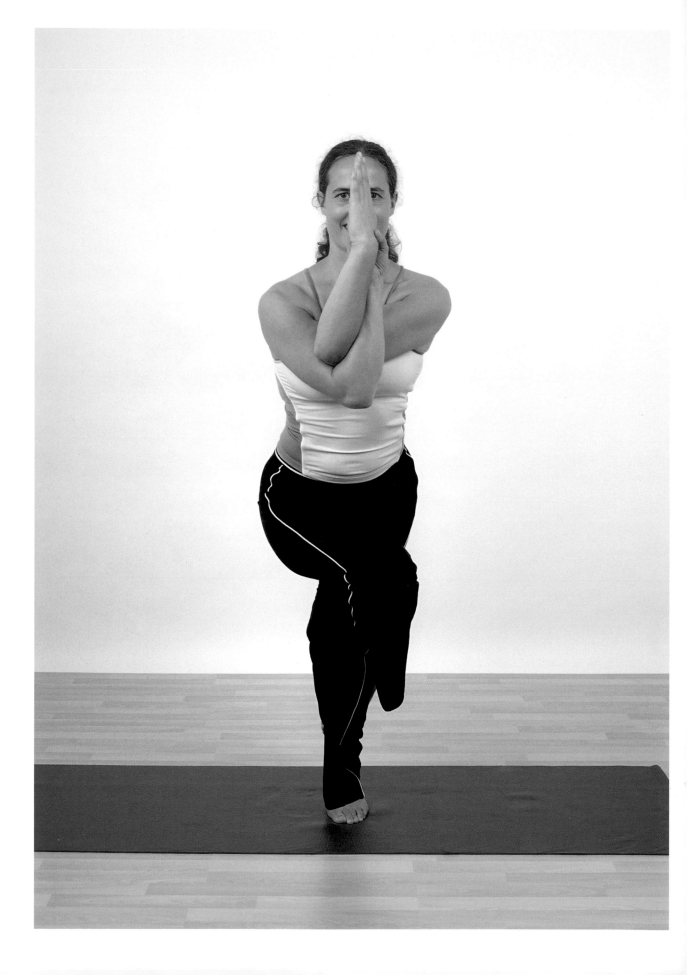

CHAPTER 2

Maintaining Healthy Joints

Warm-up stretches help to loosen the 12 primary joints in the body—both ankles, knees, hips, wrists, elbow, and shoulders, as well as warm the spine. The exercises are useful for anyone suffering from arthritis or recovering from injury. The warm-up series releases residual tension in the muscles, eases stiffness in the joints, and prepares the body for the more complex poses. On a subtle level, they also remove energy blocks, allowing prana, or energy, to move smoothly around the body, giving greater freedom of movement. It is important to perform the warm-up exercises gently and without strain, following the natural rotation of the joint. While practicing the movements, bring awareness to the interaction of the joints, ligaments, and muscles, and observe how each movement relates to other areas of the body.

Neck side stretch

Stand in *tadasana* (see page 60), or sit upright on a supportive chair. Bend and lift the right elbow and place the right hand on the left side of the head, with the elbow pointing to the side as shown. Inhale. Exhale, gently pulling the head to the right toward the right shoulder. Keep the head facing forward, and make sure that the left shoulder stays relaxed and down. Hold the position for a few seconds, breathing evenly, then repeat it on the opposite side.

BENEFITS The neck movements tone all the nerves that pass through the neck and are connected to the different parts of the body. Practicing them can help relieve stiffness and tension from the neck and shoulders.

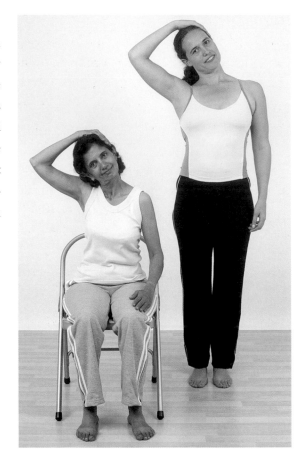

Head turns

1. Stand in *tadasana* (see page 60) or sit upright on a chair, and inhale. Exhale and turn the head to look over the left shoulder. Hold for a few moments, breathing evenly.

2. Inhale, turn back to the center and repeat on the other side.

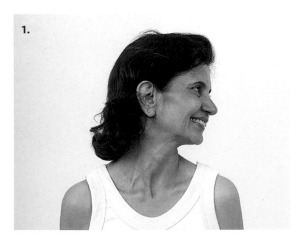

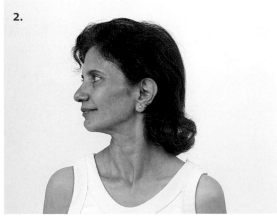

Head rolls

1. Practice the steps of this asana as one flowing movement. Begin by standing or sitting upright in a comfortable seated position, with the arms and shoulders relaxed. On an exhalation, lower the chin toward the sternum.

2. On an inhalation, gently roll the head up and to the side to look over the right shoulder. Make the movement as soft and fluid as possible. Continue to roll the head up on the inhalation to look up toward the ceiling. Make sure that the shoulder blades relax down the back.

3. Exhale, slowly drop the head to the opposite side to look over the left shoulder, then roll the head back to the first position. Repeat the exercise twice in each direction. If you feel discomfort in the neck, rest in that position for a moment or two and breathe into the area to release the tension.

1.

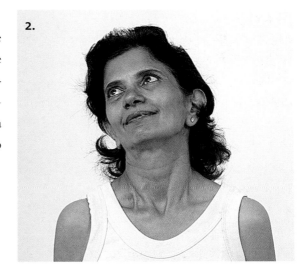

2.

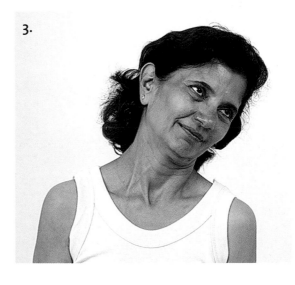

3.

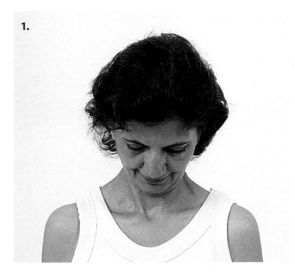

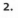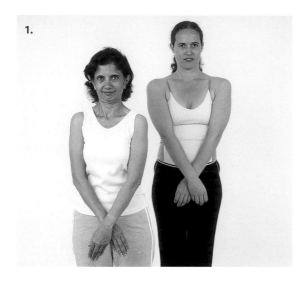

Shoulder circles

1. Stand in *tadasana* (see page 60) with the feet together. Make loose fists with the hands and cross the arms at the wrists.

2. Inhale and slowly rotate the arms up and over the head. Make sure that the shoulders stay relaxed.

3. Continue the rotation on an exhalation, allowing the arms to naturally move out to the sides. Rotate the arms back and out to the sides, moving all the way around and back to the starting position. Repeat the rotation at least twice in one direction, and then twice in the opposite direction. When you circle the shoulders in the opposite direction, rotate the arms backward and cross the wrists above the head to come forward.

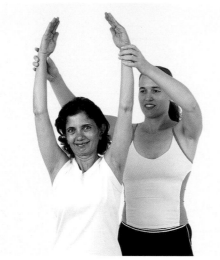

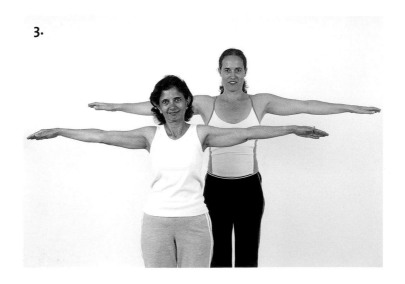

Elbow bends

1. Stand or sit upright in a comfortable seated position, with the arms and shoulders relaxed. Inhale, bend the elbows and place the hands or fingertips on the shoulders.

2. Exhale, straighten the elbows, and extend the arms forward. Repeat 3 to 5 times.

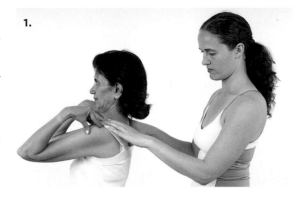

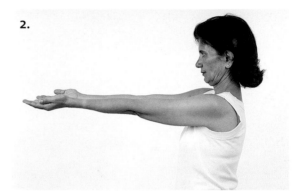

Wrist rotations

Stand or sit upright in a comfortable seated position, with the arms and shoulders relaxed. Lift the arms to an easy position and gently rotate the hands in a circular motion, 10 times in one direction and then 10 times in the opposite direction.

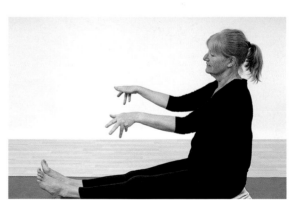

Ankle rolls

Sit in *dandasana* (see page 79) with the legs outstretched. Lift the right leg a few inches from the floor and gently circle the foot, holding the leg as shown. Rotate 10 times in one direction and then 10 times in the opposite direction. Repeat with the other leg.

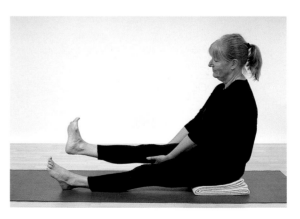

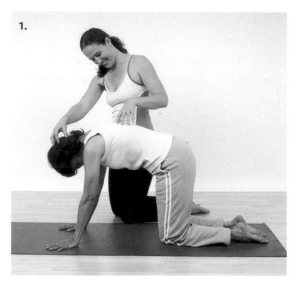

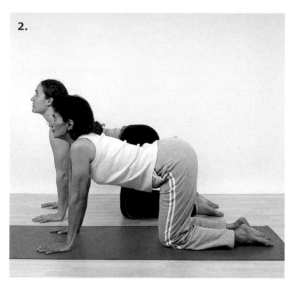

Cat pose *Majariasana*

This pose warms and limbers the whole spine. Initiate movement from the base of the spine.

1. Start on all fours, with hands beneath the shoulders and the knees beneath the hips. Inhale, lift the tailbone, concave the spine, and drop the belly. Press the hands into the floor, lift the chest and head, and look up.

2. Exhale, tuck the tailbone under, arch the back, and roll your head under, moving the chin toward the chest. Stretch the spine as high as you can. Curl the tailbone under. Repeat steps 1 and 2 for a few rounds. Make the movements as fluid as possible in time with the breath.

Eagle pose *Garudasana*

1. Stand in *tadasana* (see page 60). Focus on a spot in front of you for balance. Inhale, and raise the arms over the head.

2. Exhale as you release your arms, passing the right arm under the left arm.

3. Twist the arms around each other and touch palms. Bend the elbows so the palms are in front of the nose. Inhale.

4. Exhale, bend the knees and lift the right thigh over the left thigh. Wrap the right foot around the left calf. Try to keep knees and elbows in one line in the center of the body. Hold for 8 seconds, breathing evenly. Release and repeat on the opposite side.

BENEFITS   Eagle pose strengthens the ankles and calves, removes stiffness in the hips and shoulders, improves circulation, and develops concentration and balance.

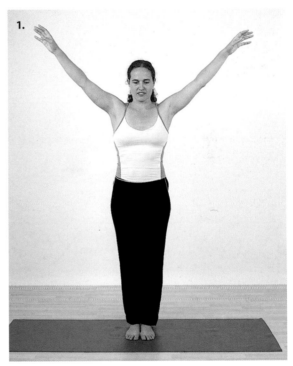

1.

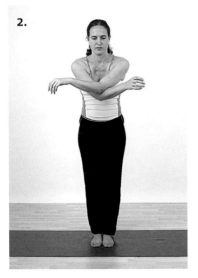

2.

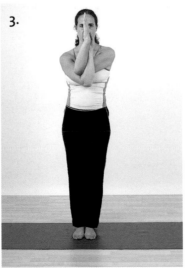

3.

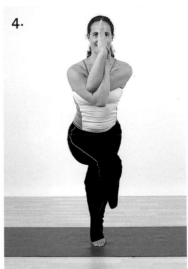

4.

Sun salutation *Surya Namaskar*

Surya Namaskar is a dynamic series of 14 asanas that are linked together with the breath. The flow of asana acts as a complete body warm-up that creates heat in the body, which limbers the spine and tones the joints, muscles, and internal organs.

1. Stand in *tadasana* (see page 60) at the front of the mat with the feet together, and the palms touching in front of the chest.

2. Inhale and stretch the arms up over the head and look toward the thumbs. Lift the chest up and gently arch the back. Keep the arms alongside the ears. Be careful not to strain the lower back.

3. Exhale and bend forward from the hips, keeping the back and legs straight and the arms extended.

4. Bend the head down toward the knees and place the hands on either side of the feet. If the hands do not touch the floor, bend the knees.

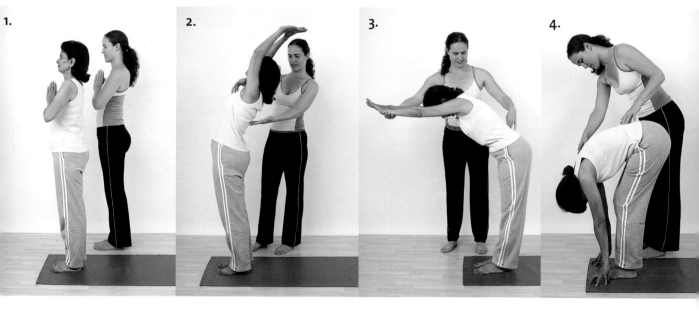

5. Inhale and stretch the right leg far back and drop the right knee to the floor. Lift the chest, and look up.

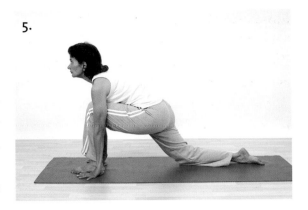

6. Exhale and step the left foot in line with the right. Come into a downward facing dog by pushing into the hands, lifting the pelvis up and back, and stretching the heels toward the floor. Relax the head and neck and look toward the feet. Inhale.

7. Exhale, bend the knees to the floor and the elbows backward; lower the chest to the floor, leaving the pelvis raised. Place the chin on the floor.

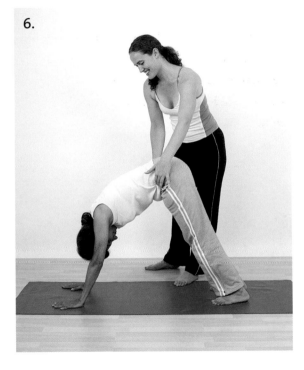

8. Inhale, drop the pelvis, tuck the tailbone under and slide the body forward, lengthening the spine. Lift the head, neck, and chest without too much pressure in the hands. Look up. Keep the pelvis on the floor.

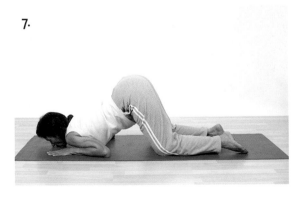

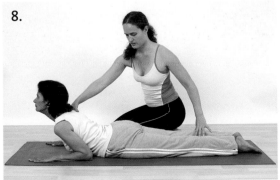

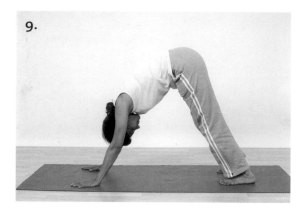

9. Exhale and push into the hands, raising the buttocks and back into downward dog pose, so that the body forms a triangle. Relax the crown of the head toward the floor and release the neck. Keep lengthening the spine and take the heels to the floor.

10. Inhale, step the right foot forward, in line with the hands. Lower the right knee to the floor, lift the chest, lengthen the spine, and look up.

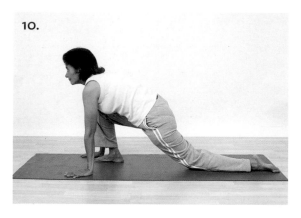

11. Exhale. Step the left foot forward in line with the right foot, coming into a forward bend. Lift up the pelvis and straighten through the backs of the knees. Relax the head toward the knees.

12. Inhale, stretch the arms forward alongside the ears, elongate the spine, lift the torso, and return to standing with the arms raised over the head.

13. Lift the chest and gently arch the back.

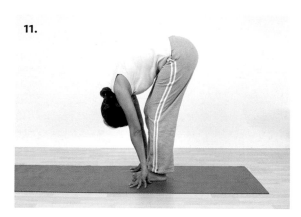

14. Exhale and bring the hands into prayer position in front of the chest. Repeat the cycle leading with the left foot to complete one full round of *Surya Namaskar.*

12.

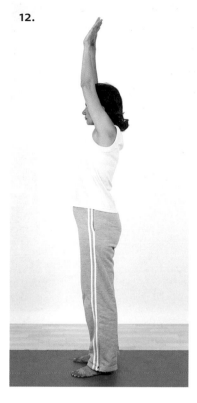

13.

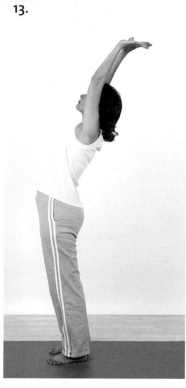

14.

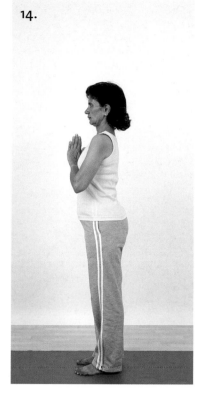

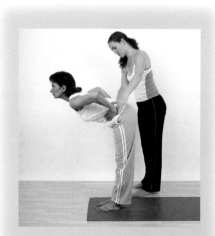

✳ **TIP** If you are suffering from a lower back problem then bend the knees and place the hands on the hips to move in and out of the forward bends, steps 4 and 12.

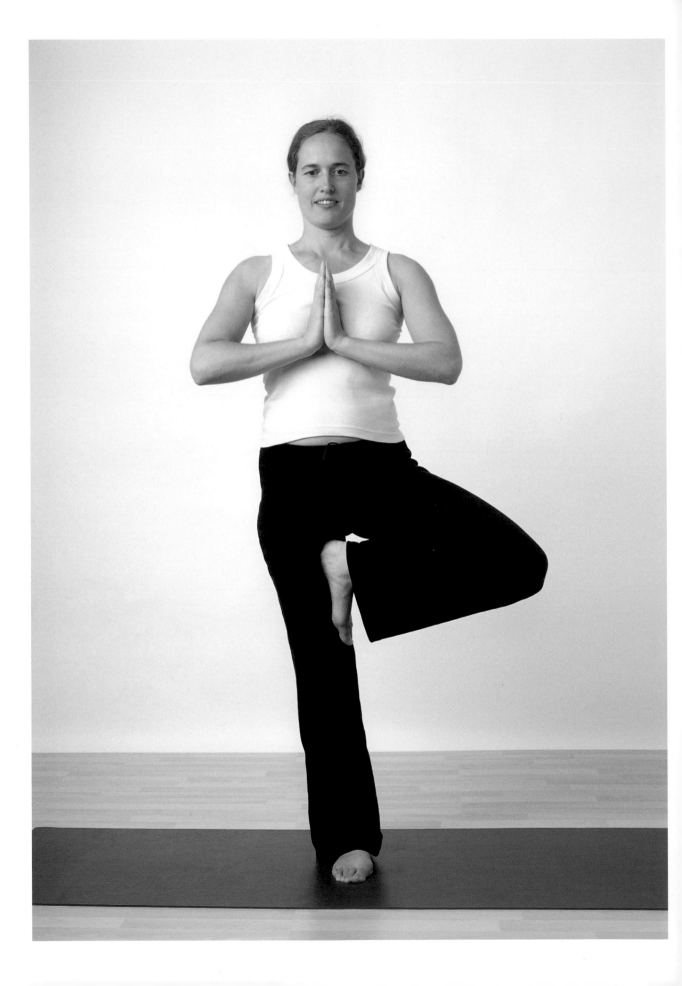

CHAPTER 3

Standing Poses

ೕ

The standing poses help to build a strong and stable foundation starting from the feet upward, as well as improving balance and coordination. More importantly, they teach us to stand on our own two feet, building confidence, poise, and grace. A refreshing tonic for the entire body, standing poses stimulate breathing, improve the circulation, aid the digestive system, and improve our mobility; they are particularly beneficial for those suffering from arthritis and rheumatism. Standing poses act as further warm-up exercises because they warm the larger muscle groups of the body with their larger movements. Due to the rotational and bending motion of the standing poses, the major joints of the body are lubricated and the skeletal structure is realigned. For safety, remember always to practice these poses on a non-slip surface.

Mountain pose *Tadasana*

Tadasana is the primary standing pose that teaches realignment and balance, and steadies the mind. Return to tadasana between each standing pose.

1. Stand with the feet together and spread the toes. Stand straight, with the spine elongated and the chest lifted. Distribute the weight evenly on both feet. Keep the legs strong and lift the knees up by pulling up the thigh muscles. The head, shoulders, and hips should be directly over the ankles with the tailbone tucked under slightly. Keep the arms extended along the sides of the body, with the hands relaxed.

2. Roll the shoulders forward and back, so the shoulder blades relax down the back. Tuck the chin in slightly, extending the back of the neck. Feel the lower half of the body from the navel down rooted into the ground, and feel the upper body from the navel up lifting toward the heavens. Breathe evenly for 8 or more breaths.

1.

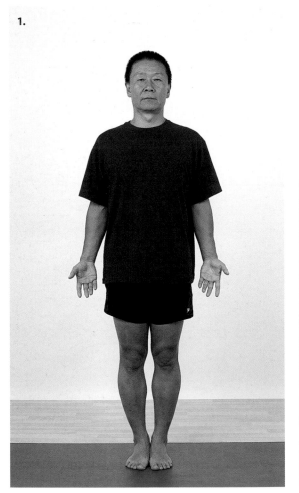

2.

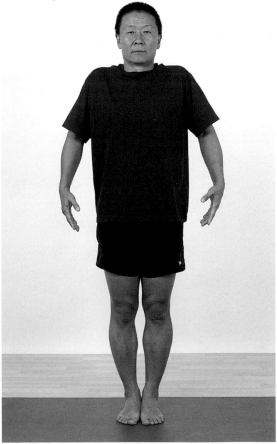

Raised-arm mountain pose
Urdhva Hastasana

1. Stand in *tadasana* (see opposite). Inhale and extend the arms out to the sides and up until the arms are parallel overhead.

2. Straighten through the elbows and look up. Breathe evenly for 8 breaths. Release the arms.

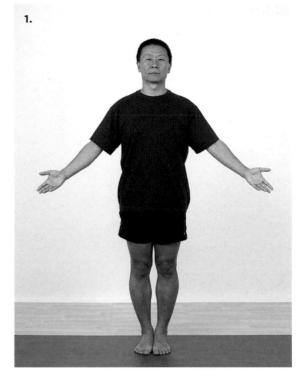

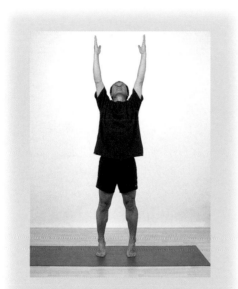

✳ **TIP** This variation helps to stretch and strengthen the toes. Stand with the feet hip-width apart. Inhale and raise the arms overhead. Push down through the balls of the feet and rise up on to tiptoes. Stretch up for 8 breaths.

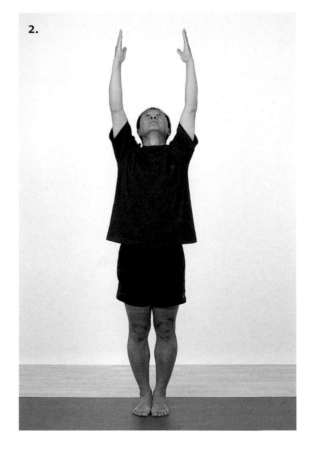

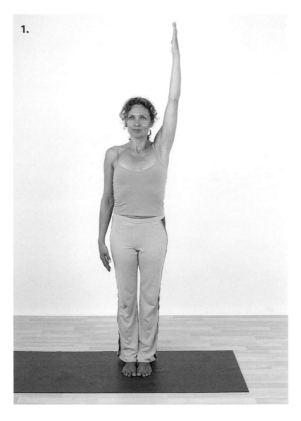

1.

Standing side stretch *Tiryaka Tadasana*

1. Stand in *tadasana* (see page 60). Inhale and raise the left arm up, alongside the head, with the palm facing toward you.

2. Exhale, pushing the hips over to the left, lift up out of the waist and stretch the body over to the right. Feel the stretch along the left side from the heels to the toes. Do not collapse on the right side. Hold for 8 breaths. Repeat on the opposite side.

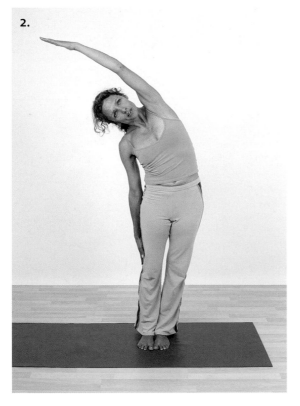

2.

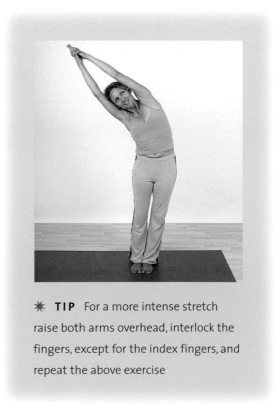

✴ **TIP** For a more intense stretch raise both arms overhead, interlock the fingers, except for the index fingers, and repeat the above exercise

Forward bend 1 *Uttanasana I*

1. Stand with the feet together and inhale. Place the hands on the hips and lift the chest. Exhale and bend forward as far as possible without bending the knees.

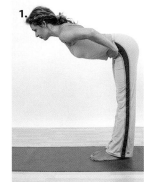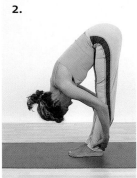

2. Clasp behind the ankles and draw the face to the knees with the hips in line with the feet. Lift up the inner arches of the feet, keep the legs strong, and relax the upper body. Hold for 8 breaths.

Forward bend 2 *Uttanasana II*

This variation releases tension in the neck and shoulders.

1. Stand with the feet together and inhale. If you have lower back pain, practice this pose with the toes turned in slightly. Clasp the hands behind the back, stretch the shoulder blades down, and lift the hands away from the buttocks.

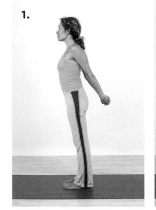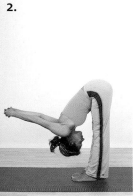

2. Exhale. Leading with the chest, bend forward from the hips and take the head toward the knees. Soften the shoulders, release the arms, and stretch the hands away.

BENEFITS   In forward bend, the heart is rested and the organs of the head receive a fresh suply of oxygen-rich blood.

✳ **VARIATION** To learn to bend forward with a straight back, stand with the feet hip-width apart. Bend forward and place the hands on the back of a chair. In this position, focus on lengthening the spine by lifting through the backs of the legs and stretching the pelvis back away from the head.

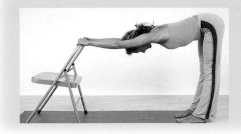

Powerful pose *Utkatasana*

Stand in *tadasana* (see page 60) with the feet hip-width apart and the outside edges of the feet parallel. Inhale and raise the arms to shoulder height, palms facing the floor. Exhale and bend the legs, as if you were going to sit down on a chair. Keep the legs parallel, shift the body weight into the heels and lift the chest. Hold for 8 breaths.

BENEFITS *Utkatasana*, powerful pose, strengthens the ankles, knees, and thighs, and shapes the legs. It reduces stiffness in the back and tones the spine.

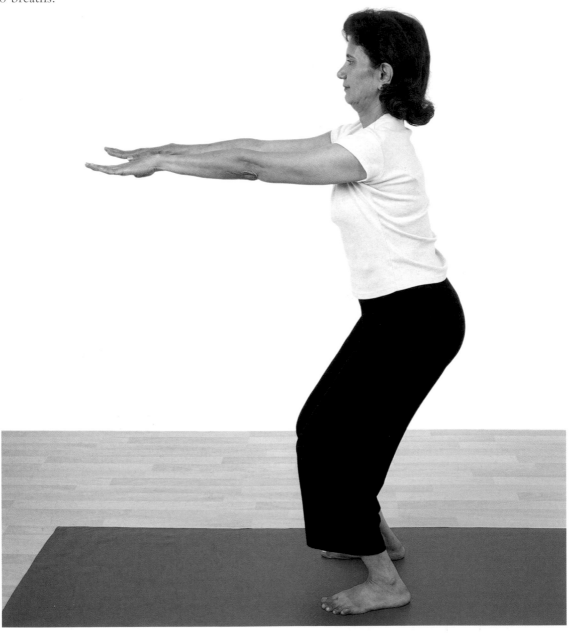

Triangle pose *Trikonasana*

1. Stand with the feet 3 to 4 feet (1 to 1.2 m) apart with the arms extended at shoulder height with the palms facing the floor. Relax the shoulders and pull the kneecaps up by tightening the thigh muscles. Turn the right leg out so that the right foot points toward the end of the mat, keeping the knee in line with the ankle. Turn the left foot in slightly toward the right side, the instep in line with the right heel.

2. Inhale and on exhalation bend to the right, placing the right hand on the ankle or as far down the leg as you can reach. Stretch the left arm up and turn the head to look up. Keep the left hip lifted and rotate the chest so that the body is in one plane. Breathe steadily for 8 breaths. Repeat on the left side.

BENEFITS *Trikonasana* improves flexibility in the spine, and alleviates back and neck pain. It massages and tones the pelvis and abdomen, relieving indigestion and gas.

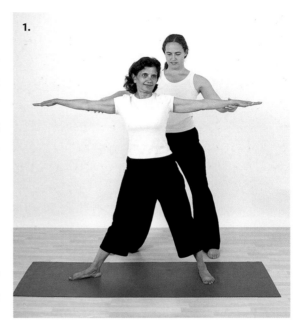

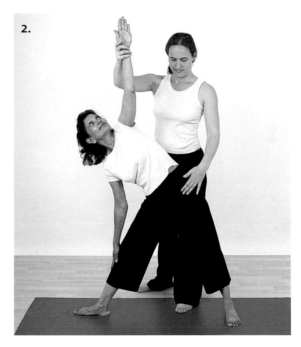

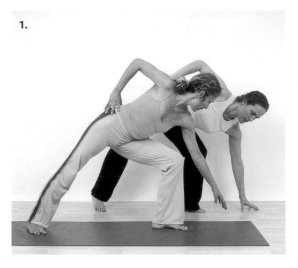

Half-moon pose *Ardha Chandrasana*

1. Step the feet 3 to 4 feet (1 to 1.2 m) apart. Turn the left leg and foot out toward the end of the mat and turn the back foot in slightly. Place the right hand on the right hip. Exhale, bend the left knee and bend sideways, placing the hand on the floor about 1 foot (30 cm) from the front foot. Inhale.

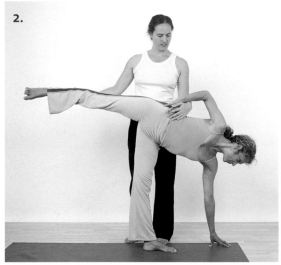

2. Exhale and draw the back foot in, straighten the left leg and lift the right leg up until it is parallel with the floor. Rotate the chest and lift the right hip so that the body is on one plane.

3. Extend the right arm so that both arms form a straight line. Stretch into the heel of the left leg and look up at the right thumb. Maintain the weight in the standing leg, not the arm. Breathe steadily 8 or more times, then repeat the pose on the other side.

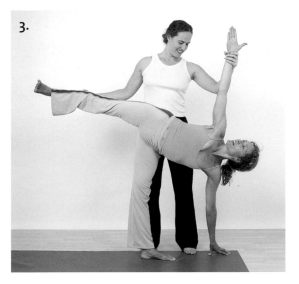

BENEFITS *Ardha chandrasana,* improves concentration and balance, bringing agility and lightness to the body, and relieves backache and sciatica. The pose helps to correct a prolapsed uterus.

Extended side stretch *Parsvakonasana*

1. Step the feet 4 to 4½ feet (1.2 to 1.4 m) apart. Extend the arms out to the sides. Rotate the right leg and foot 90 degrees, but keep the hips facing forward and turn in the left foot slightly. Bend the right knee until it is directly over the ankle joint.

2. Inhale, then on an exhalation lean over to the right side, and place the right hand on the outside of the right foot with fingers in line with the toes. Keep the feet grounded and maintain pressure along the outside edge of the left foot. Keep the thigh of the bent leg parallel to the edge of the mat and the knee at a right angle. Rotate the left arm until the palm is facing up, then extend it alongside the left ear, forming a diagonal line along the left side of the body from the heel to the fingertips. Turn the head and look up. Breathe evenly for 8 breaths. Repeat the pose on the opposite side.

1.

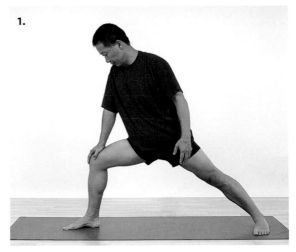

2.

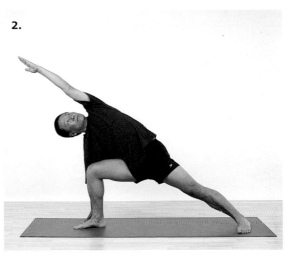

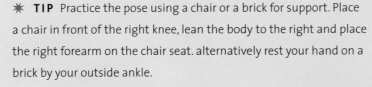

✳ **TIP** Practice the pose using a chair or a brick for support. Place a chair in front of the right knee, lean the body to the right and place the right forearm on the chair seat. alternatively rest your hand on a brick by your outside ankle.

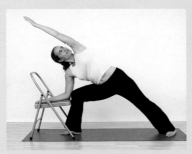

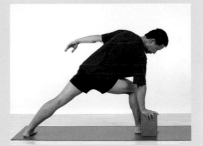

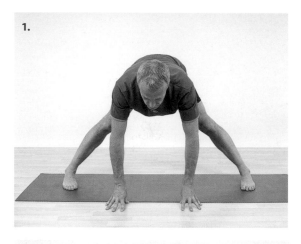

Extended leg pose *Padottanasana*

1. Step the feet 4 to 4½ feet (1.2 to 1.4 m) apart and place the hands on the hips. With the feet parallel and the legs strong, bend forward with a flat back, placing the hands on the floor directly under the shoulders. Keep the hips in line with the heels and extend the torso from the pelvis to the crown of the head. Breathe 8 times.

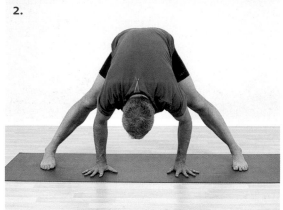

2. Exhale, walk the hands in line with the feet. Take the head toward the floor between the hands. Relax the body and keep the legs strong. Maintain the pose for 8 breaths.

> ✳ **TIP** For beginners, place the hands on blocks in Step 2 and focus on elongating the spine.

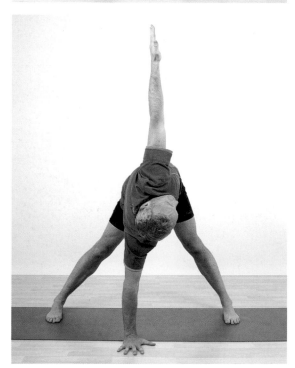

Extended leg pose twist

Parivrtta Padottanasana

Step the feet 4 to 4½ feet (1.2 to 1.4 m) apart and place the hands on the hips. Keep the feet parallel and the legs strong. Bend forward with a flat back and place the right hand on the floor, centered between your legs. Raise the left arm and rotate the chest to the left. Look up toward the raised hand. Hold for 8 breaths, then return to the center and repeat on the opposite side.

Sideways extended pose

Parsvottanasana

1. Step the feet 3½ feet (1 m or so) apart, placing the right foot forward. Turn the right foot and leg toward the end of the mat.

Lift up onto the ball of the left foot and turn the left foot in line with the right. Rotate the hips to face forward. Place the hands on the hips and extend the spine, and inhale.

2. Exhale and extend forward over the right leg. Place the hands down on the floor alongside the right leg. Bend the head toward the right leg. Hold for 8 breaths. Repeat on the opposite side.

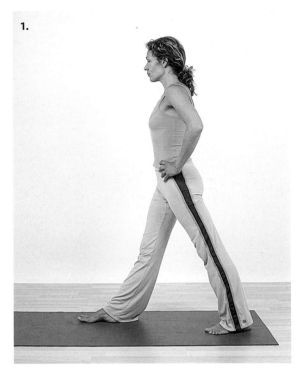

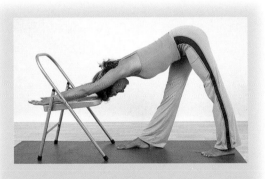

✳ **TIP** If you have difficulty bending to the floor, you can use a chair to help with this exercise.

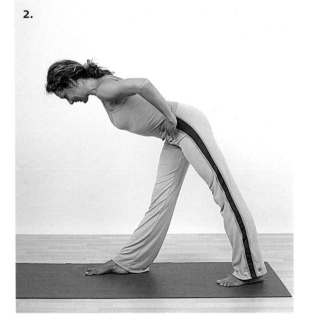

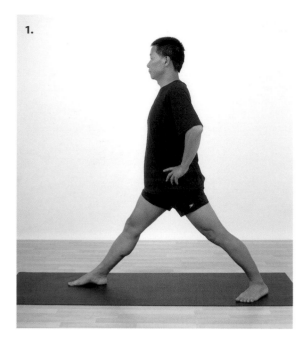

1.

Warrior pose 1 *Virabhadrasana I*

1. Step the feet 4 to 4½ feet (1.2 to 1.4 m) apart. Place the hands on the hips and then turn both feet and the hips to the right, to face the end of the mat. Inhale.

2. Raise the arms over the head into prayer position. Bend the right knee to form a right angle, lift the chest and look up. Hold for 8 breaths. Repeat on the opposite side.

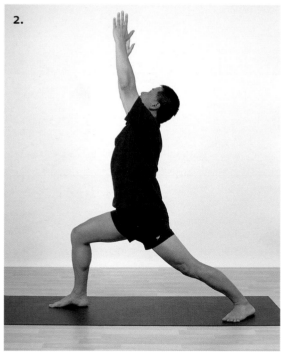

2.

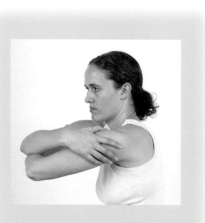

✳ **TIP** As a counter stretch to Warrior 2 (a stretch in the opposite direction to the muscles worked in the pose) place the hands on the opposite shoulders and stretch into the back between the shoulder blades.

Warrior pose 2 *Virabhadrasana II*

1. Step the feet 4 to 4½ feet (1.2 to 1.4 m) apart. Turn the right foot and leg to face the end of the mat and turn the left foot in. Extend the arms at shoulder height with palms down. Inhale.

2. Exhale. Bend the right knee to form a right angle, with the knee directly over the ankle. Keep the torso upright, and turn the head to look over the right shoulder.

3. Hold the pose for 8 breaths, then repeat on the opposite side.

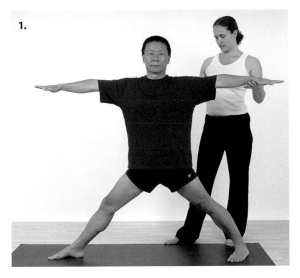

1.

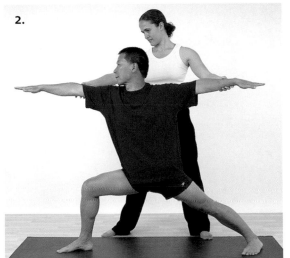

2.

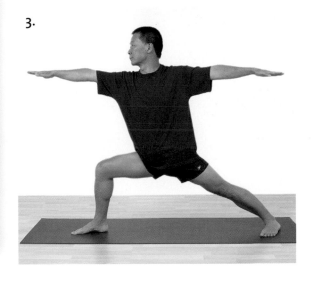

3.

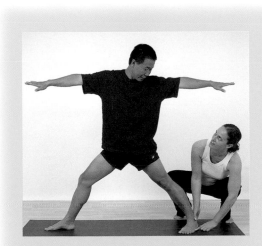

✳ **TIP** Check the position of the non-leading foot, ensuring that it stays turned inward as you move through the pose.

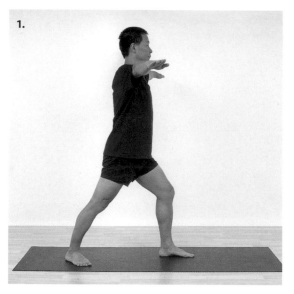

1.

Warrior pose 3 *Virabhadrasana III*

1. Stand at the end of the mat. Inhale and extend and lift the arms out to the sides. Step forward with the left leg, lean forward, and as you do this shift the body weight into the left leg.

2. Now exhale and simultaneously lift up the right leg and the back to form a straight line running from the crown of the head to the toes. Keep the hips on one plane and the head in line with the spine. Breathe 8 times, then repeat the pose on the opposite side.

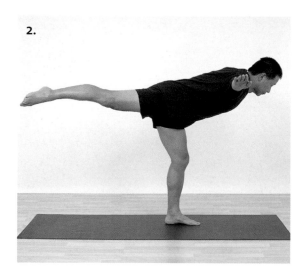

2.

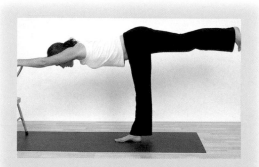

✳ **TIP** Try this pose using a chair for support. Place a chair with the back toward you about 4 feet (1.2 m) in front. (Make sure that the chair is placed on the mat as shown, or against a wall, so that it will not slip.) Bend forward and place the hands on top of the back of the chair. Raise the right leg up until it is parallel to the floor. Keep the hips level, in line with the raised leg. Hold for 8 breaths. Repeat on the opposite side.

Tree pose *Vrksasana*

Stand in tadasana *(see page 60) and spread the toes. Begin to take the body weight into the left leg.*

Raise the right leg and place the sole of the foot on the inside of the left thigh, pressing the muscle of the right leg against the left foot for support. Bring the palms together in front of the chest.

Hold for 8 breaths. To help with balance, pick a spot to concentrate on, either on the wall or about 4 feet (1.2 m) in front on the floor, or practice the pose with your back against the wall. Keep the breathing smooth and steady.

If you find that it is difficult to raise the leg as far as the inner thigh, place it either on the stationary foot or on the inside of the stationary knee. Use a chair or a wall for additional support.

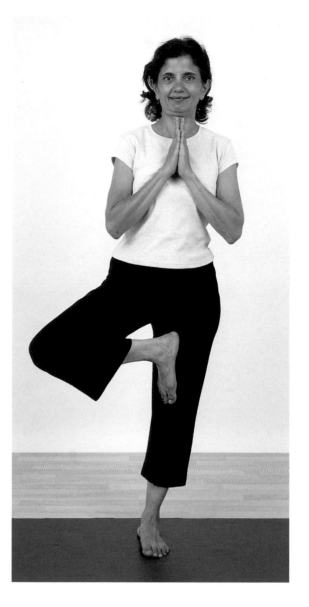

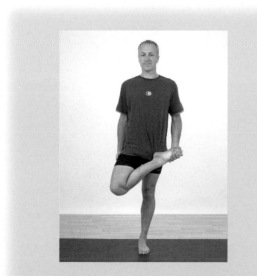

✳ **TIP** For an increases hip stretch bend the right leg and place the right ankle on top of the left thigh. Hold the right foot and rotate the right knee toward the floor. Hold for 8 breaths. repeat on the opposite side.

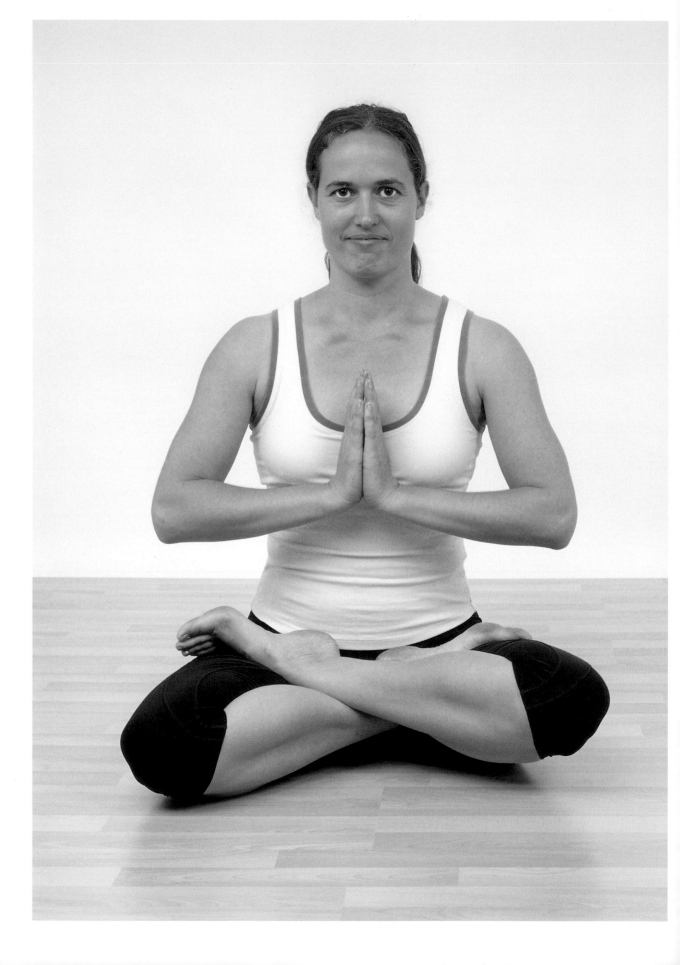

CHAPTER 4

Hip Openers

 භ

Falling is one of the greatest risks in later life, although older people who keep mobile are less likely to fall. The hip, which is essentially a ball-and-socket joint, is the largest joint in the body. Maintaining flexibility in the hips is key to remaining mobile. The following poses flex and open the hip joint. The forward bends also provide traction, creating space between the vertebrae of the spine, supplying a fresh supply of oxygen and blood to the discs, and toning the back. The following poses are suitable to practice during menstruation and menopause, and they also help regulate hormone production. Do not strain in the poses; relaxation is the key to their accomplishment.

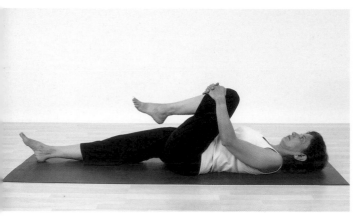

One knee to chest

Ardha Supta Pawanmuktaasana

Lie on your back with the feet together. Raise the left leg and bend the knee. Interlock the fingers around the shin. Inhale and on an exhalation, hug the bent leg close to the chest. Try to work the tailbone down toward the floor. Relax the head and neck and make sure that there is no tension in the jaw. Breathe 8 or more times. Repeat on the other side.

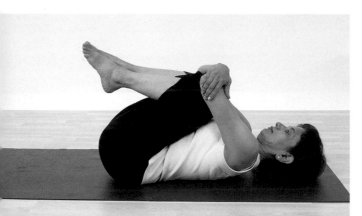

Both knees to chest

Supta Pawanmuktaasana

Lie on your back with the legs together. Bend both legs up toward the chest. Wrap the arms around the shins and on an exhalation, hug both knees closer in to the chest. As a counter stretch, curl the tailbone back down toward the floor. Keep the head and face relaxed. Hold for 8 breaths, then release the pose.

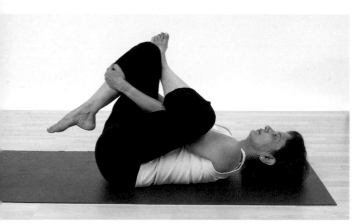

One knee to side

Supta Pawanmuktaasana

Lie on your back with the feet together. Bend both knees and place the feet on the floor close to the buttocks. Bend the left leg and place the ankle on top of the right thigh, just above the knee. Release the left knee out to the side. Reach through the inside of the left leg with the left hand and interlock the fingers around the right shin. Inhale, and on the exhalation pull the right knee in toward the chest. Hold for 8 breaths. Repeat on the opposite side.

Lying thumb-to-foot pose

Supta Padangushtasana

1. Lie flat on your back with the legs and feet together. Bend the left leg and take hold of the big toe with the thumb, index, and middle finger of the left hand.

2. Keeping hold of the big toe, inhale and straighten the left leg up, stretching into the heel of the left foot. Keep the left shoulder down, the hips level, and the right leg strong by pushing into the ground with the right thigh. Extend the right arm out to the side with the palm down.

3. Exhale and extend the left leg out to the left side, taking the heel toward the floor. Turn the head to look over the right shoulder. Hold for 8 breaths, then repeat on the opposite side.

BENEFITS As well as creating flexibility in the hips, *supta padangushtasana* is great for releasing tension and stiffness in the lower back. It tones the reproductive organs and stimulates the digestive tract.

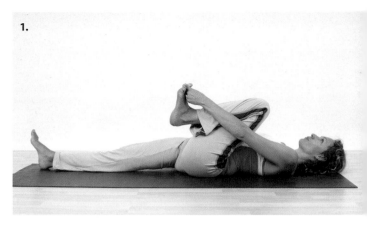

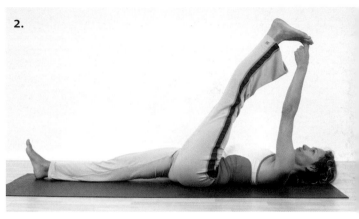

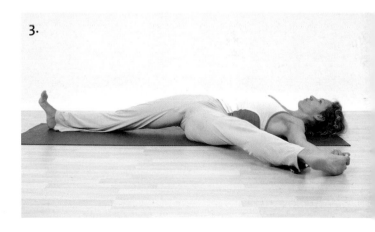

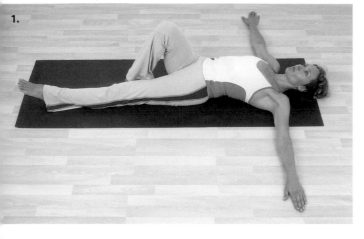

1.

Lying side stretch *Parivartanasana*

1. Lie on your back in a straight line. Extend the arms out to the side with the palms down. Bend the right knee and hook the right foot behind the left knee. Inhale.

2. Exhale and drop the right knee over to the left side. Keep both shoulders in contact with the mat. Look over the right shoulder. Relax the head, neck, and torso. Hold for 8 breaths, then repeat the pose on the opposite side.

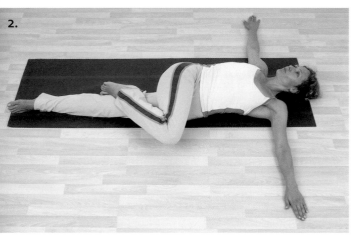

2.

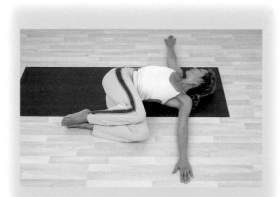

BENEFITS The twisting action of dropping the knees to the side massages and flexes the lower back, removing stiffness and tension.

✳ **TIP** For a more intense stretch, bend both knees up toward the chest. Stretch the arms out to the sides with the palms down on the floor. Inhale, then exhale and drop the knees over to the left side, revolving from the waist. Keep the right shoulder moving down toward the floor. Turn the head to look over to the right side. Relax the neck and release the back. Breathe evenly 8 or more times. Inhale, bring the legs to the center, then repeat on the other side.

Staff pose *Dandasana*

Sitting upright with the legs outstretched is called dandasana, *or staff pose. It is the neutral sitting pose for all forward bends, as is* tadasana *(see page 60) for standing poses. So between each sitting pose, come back to* dandasana.

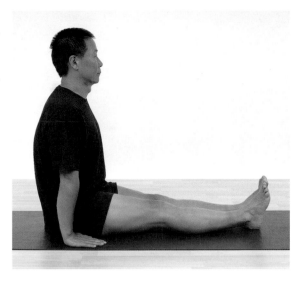

Sit upright with the legs outstretched. Keep the ankles, knees, and thighs together. Extend through the backs of the legs into the heels and draw the toes toward the head. Keep the thighs strong and pressing down into the floor. Place the palms on the floor beside the hips with the fingers extending forward. Lift up the torso from the pelvic bones; draw the abdomen in toward the spine and up toward the diaphragm. Open the chest, lift the sternum, and move the shoulder blades back and down. Tuck the chin slightly in and lengthen through the back of the neck. Keep the head, shoulders, and hips in one line. Breathe steadily for 8 breaths.

Hero pose *Virasana*

Kneel on the mat then lift the buttocks so that you are sitting on your knees. Keep the knees together and move the feet a little wider than hip-width apart, with the toes pointing backward. Slowly sit back down between the feet, easing the calf muscles out to the sides with the thumbs as you sit back. Sit up straight, lifting up from the pelvis. Hold for 8 breaths or longer, and then release.

> ✳ **TIP** If during this pose you experience any pain in your knees, or generally have difficulty sitting on the floor, take a folded blanket and place it between the feet, or rest a block under the buttocks.

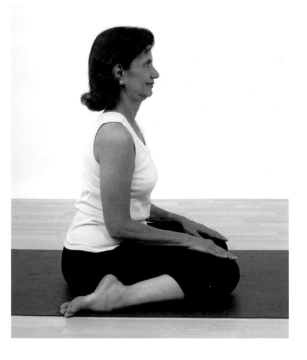

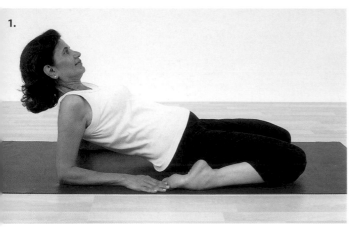

Lying hero pose *Supta Virasana*

1. When comfortable in *virasana* (see page 79) you can move on to *supta virasana*. Begin with *virasana*—inhale and exhale, reclining onto the elbows. Tuck the tailbone under. Feel the stretch through the front of the thighs and groin. Inhale, exhale, and take the upper back and head to the ground to continue the stretch.

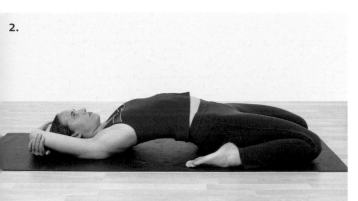

2. Tuck the chin in slightly. Stretch the arms over the head and take hold of the elbows, stretching up from waist to elbows, opening the armpits, and down from the waist toward the kneecaps. Keep both sides of the body evenly extended. There should be no knee pain as the stretch is through the front of the body. Breathe evenly 8 or more times. exhale and slowly come up.

Sage pose *Marichyasana*

In *dandasana* (see page 79) bend the left knee, placing the foot outside the right knee. Lift and turn toward the bent leg, placing the left hand behind you on the floor. Press the right thigh into the floor, extending into the heel. Breathe in, exhale, and increase the twist; wrap the right arm around the left knee. Turn the torso and the head, looking over the left shoulder. Twist up from the base of the spine turning in the hips, waist, chest, and shoulders. Hold for 8 breaths, then repeat on other side.

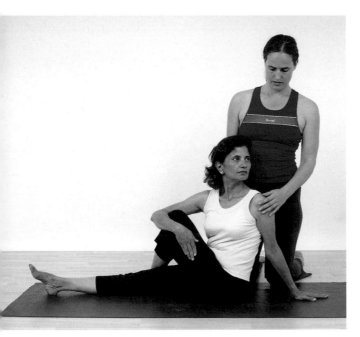

Seated forward bend *Paschimottanasana*

Sit upright in *dandasana* (see page 79). Inhale. Stretch the arms up over the head and elongate the spine. Exhale, and bend forward with a flat back over your straight legs and take the hands to the sides of the feet or as far down the leg as possible. Take the elbows out to the sides and the head toward the knees. Relax the back of the neck and shoulders. Keep the legs straight, pressing the thighs in to the floor. Hold for 8 breaths, inhale, and come up.

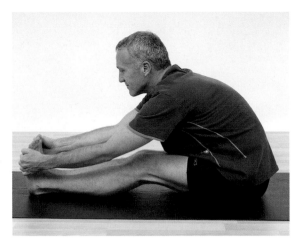

HAND VARIATIONS

Rather than touch the toes and lose a straight spine, hold the shins as you bend forward or, if you can reach the feet with a straight back, take hold of the big toes or the sides of the feet.

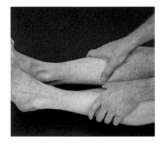 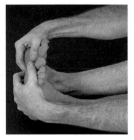

✳ **TIP** Building flexibility in the back and hamstrings requires patience and effort. If you cannot bend forward with a flat back and touch your feet, have a partner support your back or practice using a belt placed around the balls of the feet (see page 40). Only come as far forward as is comfortable without straining. As you bend forward, focus on keeping the spine erect and elongating the hamstrings.

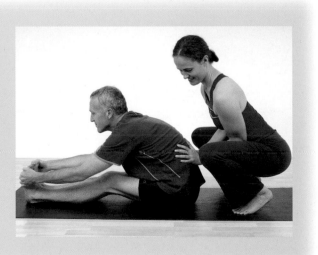

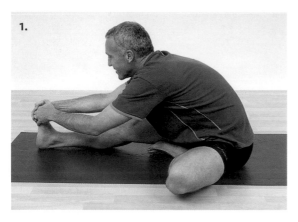

1.

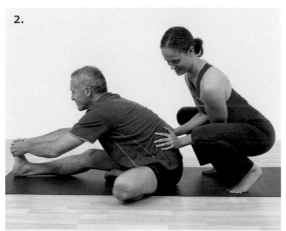

2.

Head-to-knee pose *Janu Sirsasana*

1. Sit upright in *dandasana* (see page 79). Bend the left leg and place the sole of the left foot along the inside of the right thigh. Relax the left knee down to the floor. Keep the right leg strong and extend into the right heel. Inhale, elongate the spine and raise the arms over the head. Exhale, leading with the chest, and bend forward with a flat back over the extended leg. Hold the shin, ankle, or right foot with both hands. Bend the elbows to the side to gently pull deeper into the bend. Hold for 8 breaths. Repeat on the opposite side.

2. Keep your back flat and resist letting your spine curl. Ask a partner to assist you by supporting the lower back.

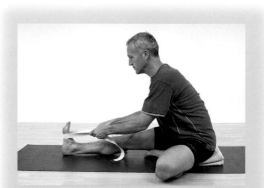

✳ **TIP** If you cannot reach the extended foot, use a belt around the ball of the extended foot (see page 40). Work on keeping the spine straight as you bend forward over the extended leg. Lift up and out of the lower back so that you pivot from the hip joints.

Rock the baby

1. Sit in *dandasana* (see page 79). Bend the right leg and take hold of the right ankle with both hands. Gently pull the ankle in and up, closer to the chest.

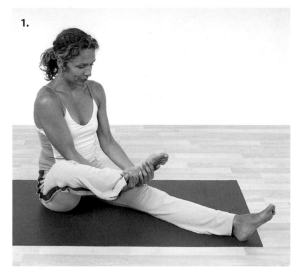

2. Place the right foot in the crook of the left arm, being careful to support the ankle joint. Wrap the right arm around the leg, placing the right knee in the crook of the right arm. Interlock the fingers around the outside of the right calf. Gently rock the right leg from side to side to open and massage the right hip joint. Continue rocking 8 to 10 times, breathing evenly. Repeat with the opposite leg.

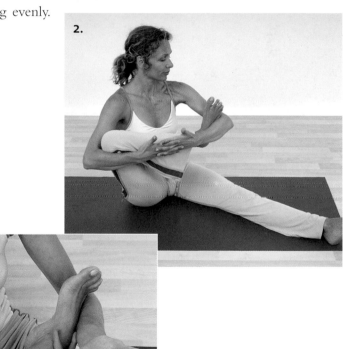

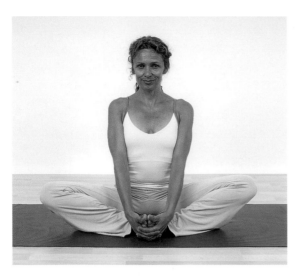

Cobbler pose *Baddha Konasana*

Sit in *dandasana* (see page 79) with the legs out-stretched. Bend both knees and bring the feet in as close to the groin as possible. Touch the soles of the feet together. Drop the knees to the sides. Hold the feet, keeping the spine straight and lifted. Hold for 8 breaths or longer.

BENEFITS *Baddha Konasana* is a gentle pose that increases mobility in the hip joint.

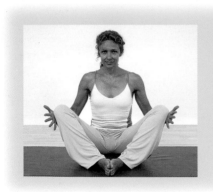

✴ **TIP** When coming out of the pose, support the knees with the hands and release slowly.

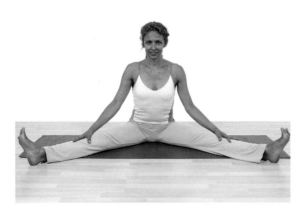

Seated angle pose *Upavista Konasana*

Sit in *dandasana* (see page 79). Stretch the legs out to the side as wide as possible. Keep the knees and feet pointing up. Press the thighs into the floor and extend into the heels. Place the hands on the legs, or the palms on the floor in front with fingers facing forward. Breathe evenly for 8 breaths.

✴ **TIP** The lower back has a tendency to sag or roll under in this pose. Place a block or folded blanket under the buttocks to lift the hips.

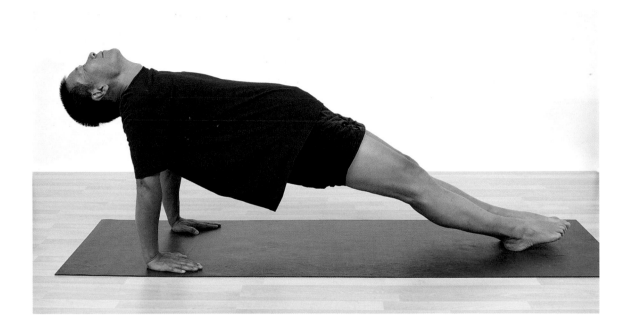

Table pose *Purvottanasana*

Purvottanasana provides the perfect counter-stretch to forward bending. It gently works the hips in the opposite direction, opens the groin, and releases tension in the lower back. Sit in *dandasana* (see page 79). Roll the shoulder blades toward the spine and to open the chest. Place the hands behind the back about 1 foot (30 cm) from the buttocks, with the fingers pointing forward. Inhale, lean into the hands, press down with both heels and lift the pelvis.

Point the toes and extend the soles of both feet onto the mat. Keep lifting up, open the chest, gently release the head and look back. Now exhale, then hold for 8 breaths, breathing evenly.

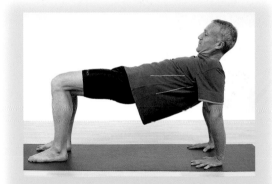

✳ **TIP** Sit in *dandasana* (see page 79). Place the hands behind the back about 1 foot (30 cm) from the buttocks. Bend the legs and place the soles of the feet on the mat, with the feet hip-width apart. Inhale, press into the hands and feet, and lift the pelvis and chest to form a horizontal line. Look forward toward the knees and hold for 8 breaths.

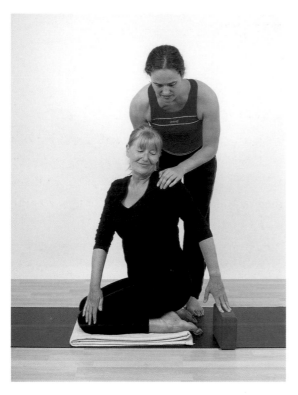

Gentle side twist

Come to a kneeling position. Inhale and extend the spine, keeping the hips, shoulders, and head in one line. Exhale, turn to the left and place the palm of the left hand on the outside of the right knee. Place the right hand on the floor or on a block behind the back. Look over the left shoulder. Keep twisting to the left, turning the navel, rib cage, shoulders and head. Breathe evenly for 8 breaths. Release the pose and repeat on the opposite side.

> ✳ **TIP** As you twist, do not allow the shoulders to lift—focus on keeping the shoulders relaxed and down.

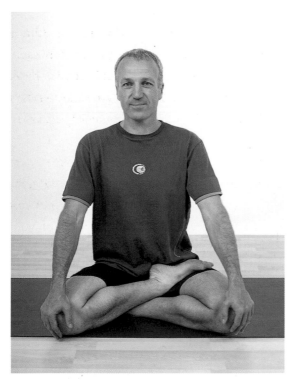

Half-lotus *Ardha Padmasana*

The half-lotus is a comfortable and safe seated pose that begins to open the hips in preparation for full lotus without straining the knees.

You can sit on a folded blanket or block to raise the hips and ease the lower back (see page 37). Sit in *dandasana* (see page 79). Bend your left leg and place the left foot close to the groin with the sole facing up. Bend the right leg and draw it close to both hands. Relax the right hip and leg completely. Lift the right foot and place it on top of the left thigh, with the sole facing upward. Sit straight with palms facing upward on your knees. Hold for 20 to 30 seconds. Release the legs and repeat on the opposite side.

Meditation

Meditation is an effective tool for managing stress because it helps to lower the level of cortisol, a hormone released by the adrenal glands in response to stress. Science has found a connection between stress and illness—when cortisol levels in the bloodstream remain too high for too long, disease can occur. Meditators have been found to have a much higher coping mechanism; they visit doctors and the hospital 50 percent less than non-meditators. The activity in the brain also changes during meditation as the brain waves become longer, akin to those produced during deeply relaxed states. The mind is gathered in the present, which cuts the natural tendency to worry about future events or obsess about previous actions. Also, meditation aids the circulation of blood to the brain, helping to keep the mind lucid in later life.

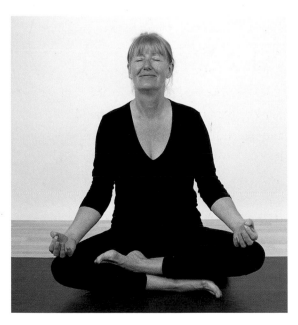

HOW TO MEDITATE

Meditation is usually practiced at the end of a yoga workout, after *pranayama* (see page 20). Like learning to play a musical instrument, meditation requires practice, for at least 20 minutes a day.

As a beginner it is important to find a peaceful spot in which to meditate that is free from external distractions such as ringing telephones or external street noise.

Find a comfortable position, either cross-legged, or in a half-lotus (see below left) or sitting on a chair with the spine upright. Wear loose-fitting, comfortable clothes and remove spectacles and watches.

It is important to maintain a passive attitude to any thoughts that arise in the mind, because initially when you sit the mind is flooded by all the activities of the day, from conversations that took place to lists of things you need to accomplish tomorrow.

Simply observe thoughts as if they were clouds floating across a clear blue sky and gently bring your awareness back to the breath or mantra. Observe the natural rhythm of your breathing, and the cool sensation as you breathe in and the warm sensation as you exhale. You can chant this mantra:

So Ham

So Ham means "I am"; say the *So* on the inhalation and *Ham* on the exhalation. Gradually with practice the mind will become more calm and peaceful.

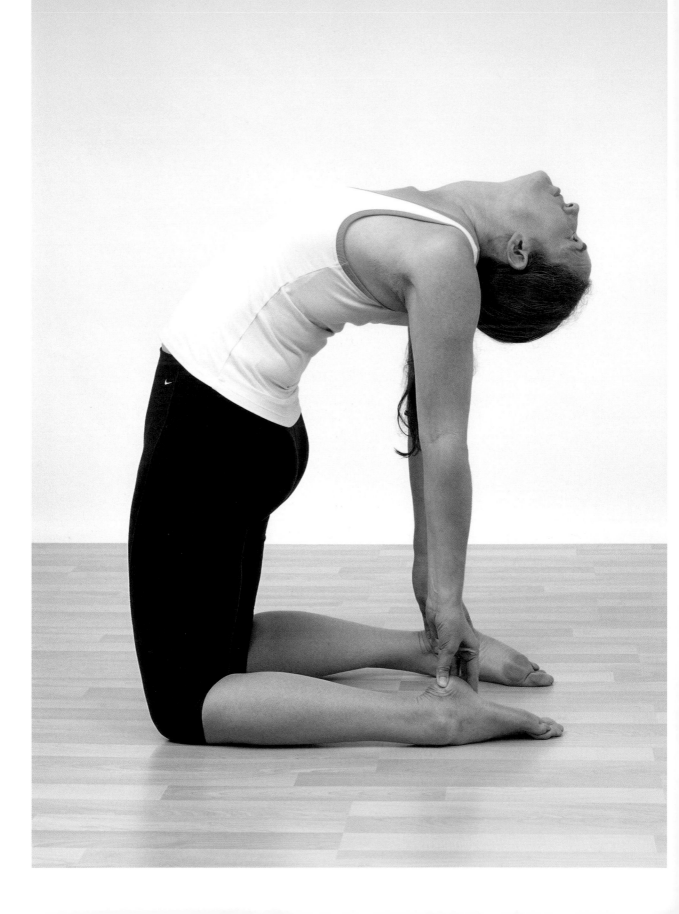

CHAPTER 5

Back-Bending

As we age, and after a lifetime of sitting at a desk, the back begins to round. A rounded spine constricts the lungs and affects our ability to breathe deeply. With less oxygen, the brain is starved and circulation deteriorates. Keeping the back strong and supple slows the aging process and keeps the body vital. Back-bending poses increase the space between the internal organs, removing toxins and allowing vital nutrients and blood to flow freely. Helpful for strengthening the muscles in the back, back-bends also flex the spine and stimulate the body's central energy channel. The following poses expand the chest and open the heart center, giving energy, courage, and mental clarity, which can help overcome depression.

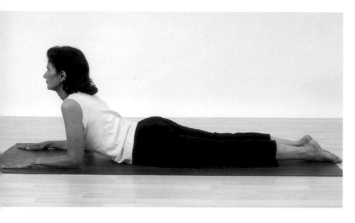

Crocodile pose *Makarasana*

Lie flat on the stomach with the feet hip-width apart. Relax the pelvis and tuck the tailbone under to lengthen the lower back. Place the hands underneath the shoulders, with the fingertips pointing forward. Place the forehead on the mat. Inhale, lift the chest and slide the forearms forward until the elbows rest directly underneath the armpits. Look straight ahead. Hold the pose for 8 breaths.

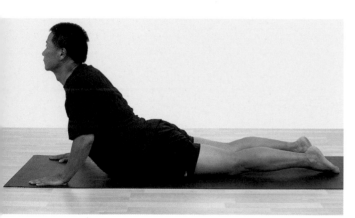

Cobra pose *Bhujangasana*

Lie flat on the stomach. Bring the feet and legs together and place the palms under the shoulders beside the rib cage. Place the forehead and then the chin on the floor. Feel the extension through the spine from the tailbone to the crown of the head. Elongate the spine, raise the head and chest and inhale. Roll the shoulders down and open the chest. Press gently into the palms, lengthening the spine vertebra by vertebra, bringing the chest forward. Keep the elbows alongside the body. Look up, without crunching in the back of the neck, and exhale. Hold for 8 breaths, breathing evenly, then exhale and release.

Half-locust pose *Ardha Salabhasana*

1. Lie face down on the mat, flat on the stomach, and place the chin on the floor. Tuck the arms under the body—have the palms either facing up or down, or make loose fists, and let them rest under the tops of the thighs.

2. Move the elbows as close together as possible. Inhale and stretch the left leg back and up. Hold for 8 breaths. Repeat on the opposite side.

> ✳ **TIP** Lift the leg as far as feels comfortable, while keeping the hip in contact with the forearm—do not force it. As you practice you will gradually be able to lift your leg higher.

1.

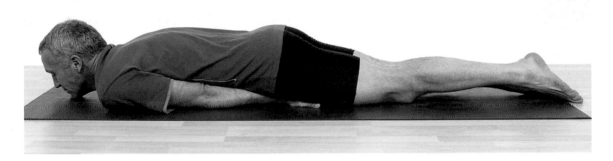

2.

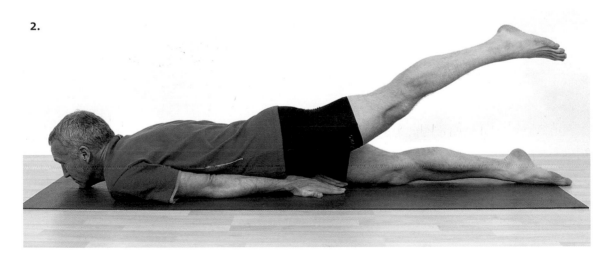

Locust pose *Salabhasana*

1. Lie flat on the stomach on the mat. Place the chin on the floor and bring the feet together. Tuck the arms under the body and shift the body weight forward into the chest and shoulders.

2. Keeping the feet and legs together, inhale, and lift both legs. Do not strain in the lower back. Hold for 8 breaths, then exhale and release the pose.

BENEFITS   *Ardha salabhasana* and *salabhasana* help to keep the back strong by strengthening the muscles of the lower back, pelvis, and abdomen. They also remove tension from the wrists and elbows, and can help alleviate the symptoms of carpal tunnel syndrome. Practicing these poses will help tone the intestines and relieve constipation.

1.

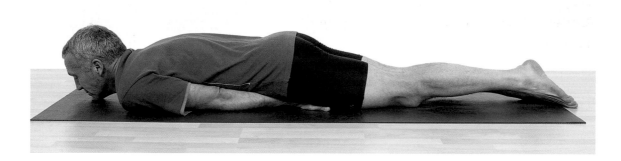

2.

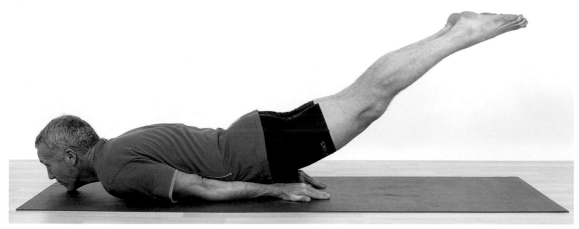

Camel pose *Ustrasana*

1. Kneel with the thighs and buttocks lifted, bringing the knees hip-width apart. Come up onto the toes. Place the hands on the lower back with fingertips pointing down, extending the spine up. Begin to lift the chest and ease the pelvis forward. Exhale as you begin to arch back.

2. Reach back one hand at a time and take hold of the heels. Keep lifting the chest.

Hold both heels and look up, without crunching in the back of the neck. Press down with the knees; keep the pelvis forward in line with the knees and the chest lifted to remove pressure from the lower back.

3. Move the shoulder blades down and into the upper back to open the chest. Extend evenly along the spine. Breathe steadily for 8 breaths. Release, holding the lower back and lifting up slowly.

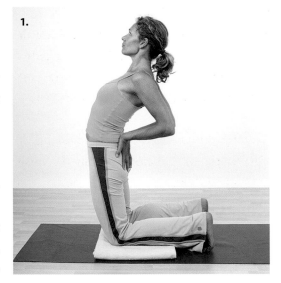

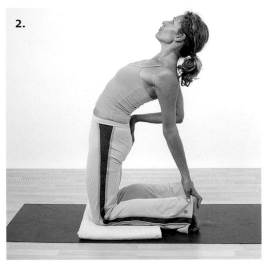

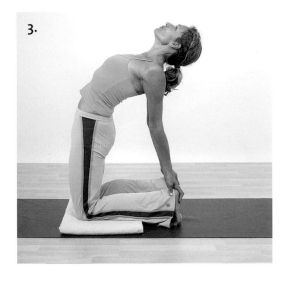

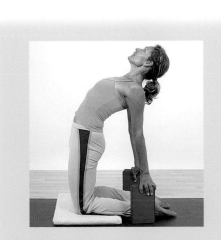

✳ **TIP** Place blocks on the outsides of the ankles. When you reach back, place the hands on the blocks for support.

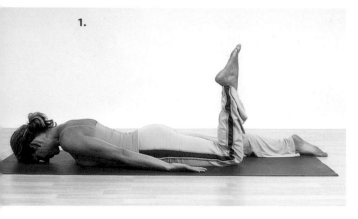

Half-bow pose *Ardha Dhanurasana*

1. Lie on your stomach, forehead on the floor and feet hip-width apart. Bend the left knee, taking the heel toward the left buttock.

2. Stretch the left arm back and take hold of the top of the left foot. Extend the right arm forward along the floor, palm down. Inhale and lift the left leg up and back. Exhale and hold for 8 breaths, breathing evenly, then repeat on the opposite side.

BENEFITS

Ardha dhanurasana flexes the entire spine, sending fresh blood and nutrients to the discs. The weight on the pelvis and abdomen tones the digestive and reproductive organs. *Dhanurasana* opens the chest, expands the lungs, and removes stiffness in the shoulders.

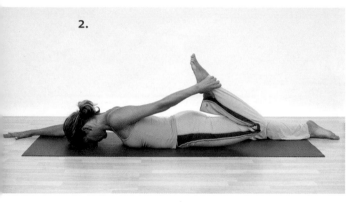

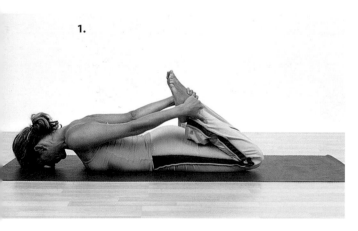

Bow pose *Dhanurasana*

1. Lie flat on the stomach. Place the forehead on the floor. Have the feet hip-width apart, bend the knees, and take the heels toward the buttocks. Stretch the arms back and take hold of the outside of the ankles. Tuck the tailbone under and place the chin on the floor. Inhale and raise the legs up and back.

2. Keep pulling up with the legs. Allow the force of the legs to lift the head and chest up as high as possible to arch the back. The spine remains passive in this pose and the shoulders relaxed.

3. Keep the arms straight as you balance on the abdomen. Raise the chin and look up without crunching the back of the neck. Exhale and breathe evenly for 8 breaths, then exhale and release the pose.

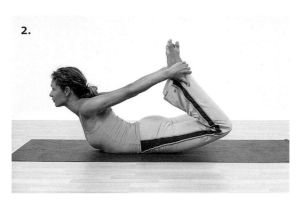

2.

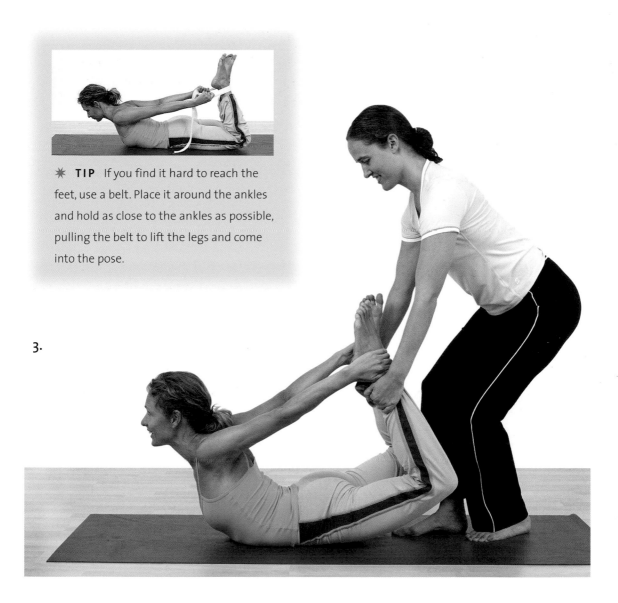

✳ **TIP** If you find it hard to reach the feet, use a belt. Place it around the ankles and hold as close to the ankles as possible, pulling the belt to lift the legs and come into the pose.

3.

Bridge pose *Setu Bandhasana*

Lie flat on your back. Bend the legs and place the soles of the feet on the floor close to the buttocks. Stretch the arms toward the feet with palms down alongside the hips.. Tuck the tailbone under. Inhale. Exhale, pushing into the palms and heels, and lift the pelvis. Roll onto the tops of the shoulders if possible and lift the chest. Tuck the chin in extending through the back of the neck. Keep the thighs strong. If comfortable, reach back with the hands and interlock the fingers. Try to keep the feet parallel—if the feet turn out, it indicates stiffness in the hips. Hold for 8 breaths. Exhale and release the pose gently, placing one vertebra at a time down onto the floor.

BENEFITS *Setu bandhasana* is a useful pose for preparing for both *chakrasana* and *sarvangasana*. It opens the shoulders and the hip joints and develops flexibility in the spine. *Setu bandhasana* is especially useful for women as it helps to regulate the menstrual cycle.

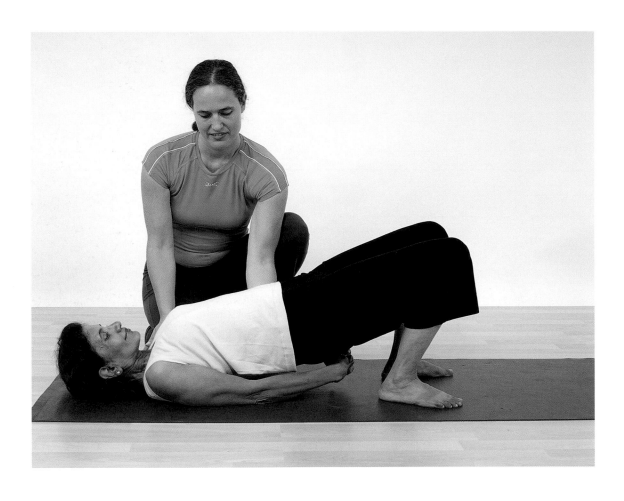

Wheel pose *Ardha Chakrasana*

1. Lie on your back. Bend the legs and place the soles of the feet on the floor close to the buttocks. Bend the elbows and place the palms of the hands flat down on the floor, underneath the shoulders. Inhale.

2. On an exhalation push into the hands and feet, raise the pelvis, and place the crown of the head on the floor. Inhale, then exhale, pushing into the palms, lifting the navel and raising the hips as high as possible. Tuck the tailbone under. Extend the chest toward the hands. Straighten the arms and keep lifting the thighs. Look down toward the floor. Breathe evenly 8 or more times, then exhale and release the pose.

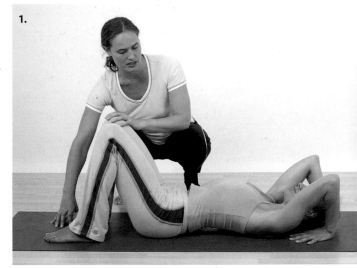

1.

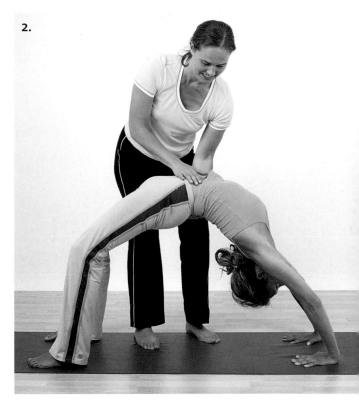

2.

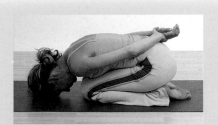

✳ **TIP** It is important after back-bending to release the spine gently in the opposite direction by coming into child's pose or gentle *paschimottanasana*.

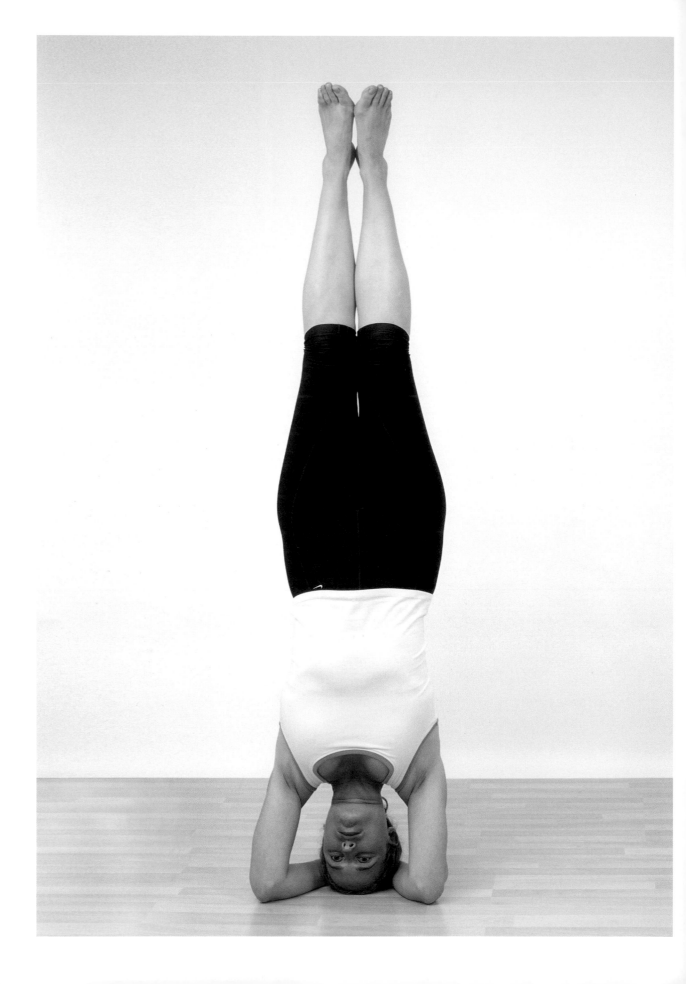

CHAPTER 6

Inversion Poses

The force of gravity asserts a constant downward pull on the body and contributes to aging. The inversions offer a welcome break and reverses the gravitational orientation of the body. Inversions send a rich supply of blood to the head and brain, which reduces wrinkles, and keeps a healthy supply of blood flowing to the brain. Turning the world upside down can help us gain a new perspective on later life. The headstand and shoulder stand are called the "king and queen of asana." because of the tremendous effect they have on the body and mind. They regulate the endocrine system, especially the pineal, pituitary, thyroid, and parathyroid glands in the head and neck, which harmonize the emotional and metabolic processes of the body by secreting hormones into the bloodstream. These inverted asanas reduce stress, anxiety, channel nervous energy, and even affect our thought processes.

Downward dog

Adho Mukha Svanasana

Lie down on the floor on your stomach. Place the palms of the hands down on the floor just below the shoulders, in line with the rib cage with the fingers pointing forward.

Make sure that the feet are hip-width apart, and tuck the toes under. Push up on to your knees. Inhale and, on an exhalation, push into the palms and raise the buttocks up and back, flattening the back of the body to form a triangle shape.

Keep the hips high and stretch the heels down to the floor, opening the backs of the knees. Look back toward the feet. Hold the pose for 8 breaths, breathing evenly, then exhale and release the pose.

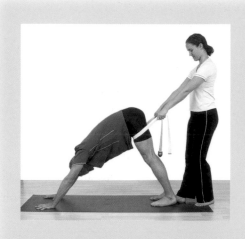

✳ **TIP** Lift the leg as far as feels comfortable, while keeping the hip in contact with the forearm—do not force it. As you practice you will gradually be able to lift your leg higher.

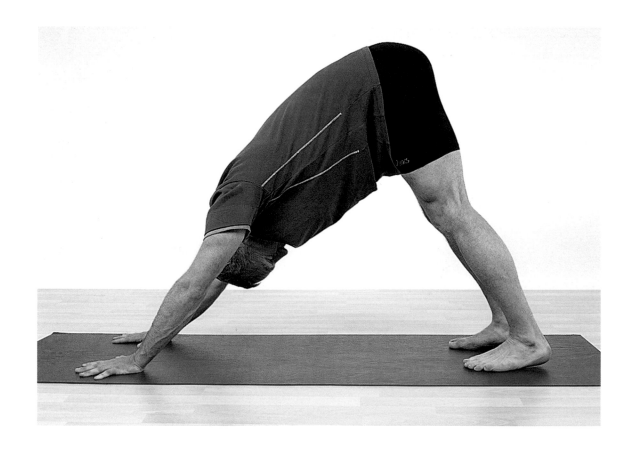

Shoulder stand with a wall

Sarvangasana

1. Lay a folded blanket close to the wall. Come into legs up the wall pose (see page 42) so the shoulder blades are flat on the blanket. Tuck the chin in, extending through the back of the neck.

2. Bend both knees and place the soles of the feet on the wall. Place arms alongside the body with the palms down, alongside the hips. Inhale.

3. Exhale, pushing against the wall with the feet and lifting the pelvis. Supporting the lower back with the hands, roll up onto the shoulder tops. Move the elbows closer for greater support.

4. Lift the feet away from the wall one foot at a time. Hold the pose for 20 to 30 seconds. To come down, bend the knees and place the feet on the wall. Exhale as you roll down one vertebra at a time.

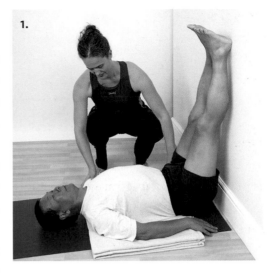

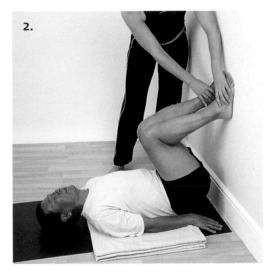

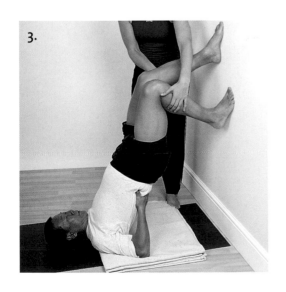

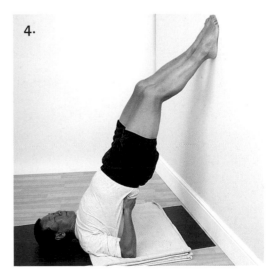

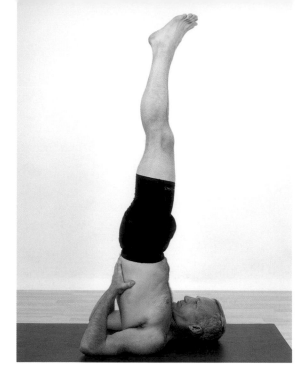

Shoulder stand *Sarvangasana*

Lie on your back. Tuck the chin in slightly and lengthen through the back of the neck. Place the arms alongside the body, with the palms down. Exhale and bend the knees, push into the palms and begin to raise the legs over the head. Bend the arms and place the hands in the middle of the back on either side of the spine to support the back without widening the elbows. Bring the torso to a vertical position, moving the chest toward the chin.

Straighten the legs to a vertical position, in line with the torso—aim for a straight line between the shoulders, hips, and ankles. Tuck the tailbone under and lengthen along the spine. Relax the muscles in the face. Inhale and breathe evenly for at least one minute. Come down or move in to *halasana*, or plow pose (see below).

BENEFITS *Sarvangasana* is the "queen" of asana: it activates the thyroid and parathyroid glands, benefiting circulation, digestion, the reproductive system, and respiration.

✳ **TIP** To come out of the shoulder stand and *halasana*, the plow, bend the knees toward the head, release the arms, and place them on the floor behind the body. Roll out of the pose, one vertebra at a time. Do not raise the head while coming out. Finally, release the legs to the floor and relax.

Plow pose *Halasana*

From *sarvangasana,* the shoulder stand, keep both legs together and exhale as you slowly lower them to the floor using strong abdominal muscles. Place the tips of the toes on the floor behind the head. The hips should be in line with the shoulders, and the backs of the thighs lifting toward the ceiling. Release the hands from the back, interlace the fingers, and stretch the arms away from the feet. Breathe evenly 8 or more times. Slowly roll out of the pose, or move on to the next variation.

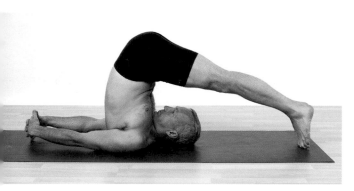

Fish pose *Matsyasana*

The fish pose should be performed after the shoulder stand as it gives a reverse stretch to the neck.

Lie on your back. Bring the legs together and tuck the hands underneath the buttocks. Push into the elbows, lift the torso, and sit up slightly to look at the feet. Lift the chest, tilt the pelvis forward, arch back, and exhale as you place the crown of the head on the floor. Relax the shoulders toward the floor. Look toward the third eye center (between the brows). Hold for 8 breaths, breathing evenly. Slowly lift out of the pose.

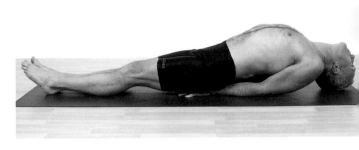

Baby headstand *Pranamasana*

1. Kneel and take hold of both heels. Tuck the chin in toward the chest and begin to curl inward, looking toward the navel. Inhale.

2. Exhale and roll forward, placing the crown of the head on the floor as close to the knees as is possible.

3. Pull on the heels and lift the hips up as high as you can; do not place too much weight on the crown. Hold for 8 breaths, breathing evenly. Exhale as you release.

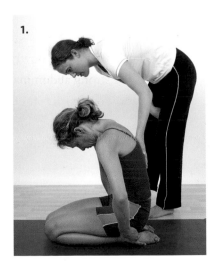
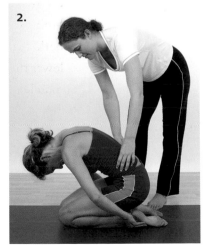
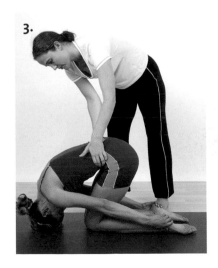

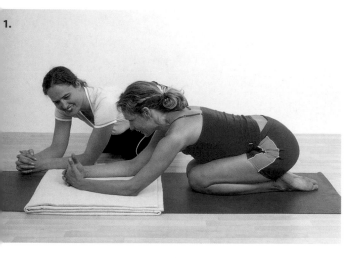

Headstand *Sirsasana*

1. From a kneeling position, place the elbows on the floor underneath the shoulders. Interlace the fingers and place the heel of the hands into the floor, with the thumb pointing up, so that the arms form an equilateral triangle. Place the crown of the head down on the floor between the hands. Straighten the legs. Breathe evenly.

2. Walk the feet forward and raise the hips in line with the head. Press the forearms down and begin to distribute the weight of the body between the arms and head. Breathe.

3. Bend the knees toward the chest and raise the feet off the floor one foot at a time. As shown, if you are not confident it can help to have a partner to assist you at this stage.

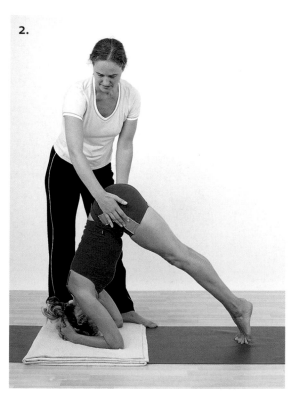

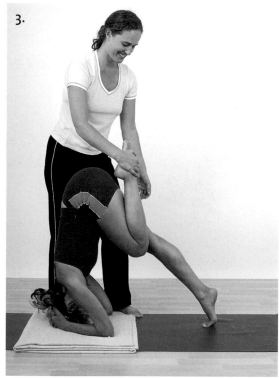

4. Inhale then exhale as you slowly extend the legs. Keep pressing into the forearms, gently lift the shoulders, and tuck the tailbone under.

5. The weight of the body should be symmetrically balanced. Relax the face and allow gravity to do the work. Breathe 8 or more times, then come down slowly.

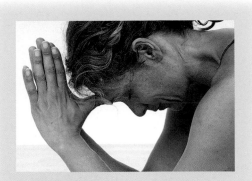

✳ **TIP** It is vital not to jump up after an inversion as the blood rushes from the head, causing dizziness. Rest in child's pose (see page 106) between inversions, or with the hands in prayer position as shown above.

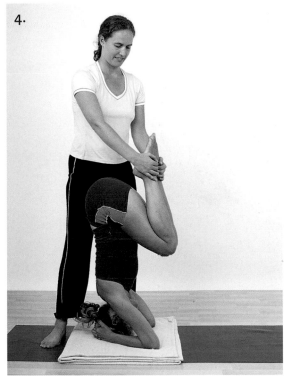

4.

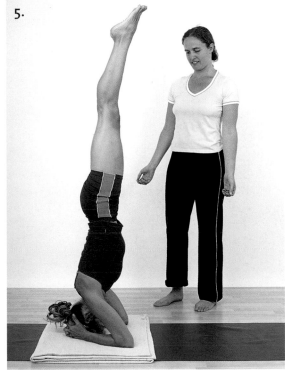

5.

Relaxation Poses

Relaxation is an integral part of yoga practice. Certain poses are considered relaxation poses and can be practiced before, after, or during a yoga *asana* session. Before practicing yoga, relaxing in either *savasana* (relaxation on the back) or *shankhasana* (child's pose) allows the body to release the stresses and strains of the day and to soothe the nervous system, preparing it for the session ahead. The same two yoga poses, along with *advasana* (relaxation on the belly) can be practiced at any point during a session if you become tired. At the end of practice it is essential to spend 10 to 15 minutes lying in *savasana*, for deep relaxation. Deep relaxation, termed *yoga nidra* or "yoga sleep," allows the benefits of the yoga *asana* session to be assimilated. *Yoga nidra* is a very difficult practice, as it is not a matter of just spacing out but rather a very conscious physical letting go while the mind remains clear and alert.

1.

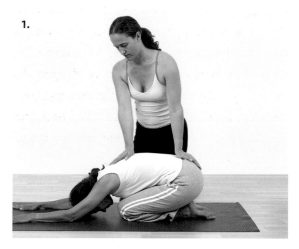

2.

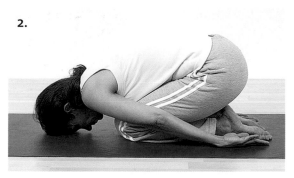

Child's pose *Shankhasana*

Child's pose can be practiced at any time, although it is particularly useful to do after back-bending to relieve tension in the lower back, or after inversions to allow time for the body to center.

1. Kneel on the mat. Slowly fold forward and place the forehead on the floor. Try to maintain the contact between the buttocks and the heels.

2. Take the arms back so that the hands are alongside the body, in line with the heels, with the backs of the hands resting on the floor. If the head does not touch the floor then place the forehead on a block. Breathe and relax the belly. Feel the abdomen pressing against the thighs on the inhale, and releasing on the exhale. Rest for a few minutes.

Relaxation on the belly *Advasana*

Resting on the belly is particularly useful between prone back-bending poses like dhanurasana *(the bow) or* salabhasana *(the locust).*

Lie on your stomach and turn the head to one side. Place the arms alongside the body, with the backs of the hands touching the floor and the palms upward. Breathe steadily, and let the belly relax. Feel the abdomen pressing against the floor on the inhalation, and releasing on the exhalation. Rest for a few minutes.

Relaxation on the back *Savasana*

During savasana *it is important not to move the body at all, as even the slightest movement creates muscular tension.*

Lie flat on the back, with the head and spine in a straight line. Move the feet about hip-distance apart and allow the feet to drop to the sides. Place the arms a few inches from the body with the palms facing up and the fingers relaxed. Tuck the chin in slightly and relax the face. Close the eyes, and allow the corners of the eyes to release and let go. Scan the body for any tension. If you observe any tension then squeeze that part of the body tightly for few moments and let go. Once the body is relaxed make a commitment not to move. Become aware of the natural breath and allow it to become rhythmic and relaxed. If the mind wanders and becomes busy then gently bring it back to the breath. Rest for 10 minutes. To come out of relaxation, begin to deepen the breath, very gently move the fingers and toes. Take a long deep stretch. Bend the knees into the chest, and roll to the right side in a fetal position. Slowly come up to stand.

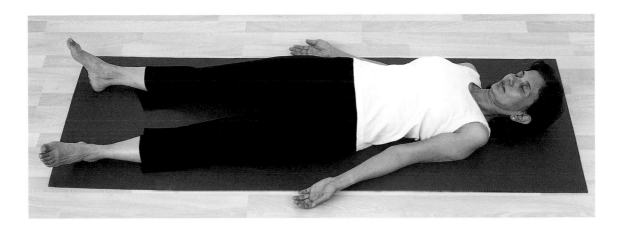

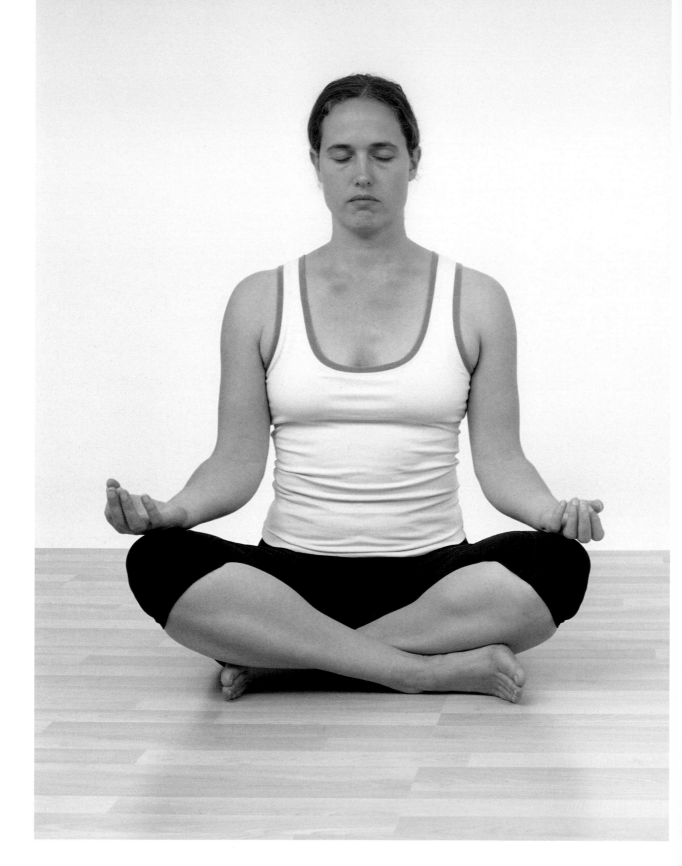

CHAPTER 7

Asanas for Ailments

Symptoms of aging, from increased body fat, stiffness in the joints and high blood pressure to brittle bones and heart disease, are not inevitable. Research indicates that age-related problems can be due to poor diet, lack of exercise, and high levels of stress. By improving your diet and taking a common-sense approach to maintaining fitness through yoga, you can become stronger, increase flexibility, have more energy, and develop a positive outlook. Yoga is unique in that the movements and techniques can be adjusted to suit each person's situation and ability. For example, during menopause the need for physically demanding yoga practice is replaced here with restorative poses to help balance the change of life. Yoga practice teaches us to "be," to become increasingly sensitive to the body and mind and release preconceived notions and expectations.

Eyes

ᘓᕽ

TO RELIEVE EYESTRAIN AND IMPROVE VISION

Age can bring changes that may weaken your eyes, making reading in particular more difficult. The eyes are designed to see a range of distances, both near and far. However, many occupations involve fixing the eyes on one plane for extended periods of time, like looking at a computer screen. The eyes are a part of the nervous system, so when the eyes become tired it creates internal stress.

Yoga recognizes the importance of caring for the eyes to maintain accurate vision and to relax the nervous system. Eye professionals agree that adequate rest and relaxation are very important for the proper care of your eyes. Stress and strain result in a build-up of pressure on the optic nerve, the eye muscles, and the retina as well as causing changes in the flow of blood in the veins that supply blood to the eyes.

Bathing the eyes in warm sunlight, by sitting with your face toward the sun with the eyes closed for 10 minutes, helps to release tension. The warmth of the sunlight will increase the flow of blood in your eyes and stimulate the nerve cells in your eyes. Diet is also important, eating plenty of vegetables and food items that contain Vitamin A, like eggs, milk, leafy vegetables, and carrots.

Yoga exercises for the eyes help to strengthen the eye muscles, tone the optic nerves, and relieve eyestrain. If practiced regularly these three exercises have been found to improve eyesight.

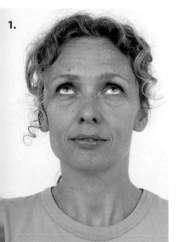
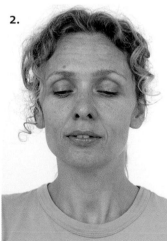

Eye exercises *Netra Vyaayaamam*
VERTICAL MOVEMENTS

1. Sit in a comfortable seated position either on a chair or on the floor. Center the eyes. Inhale, look up toward the eyebrows, without moving the head.

2. Exhale and drop the eyes to look down. Keep the vision soft and the movements fluid. Repeat 10 to 20 times. Close the eyes and rest for a few moments.

HORIZONTAL MOVEMENTS

1. Sit in a comfortable seated position either on a chair or on the floor. Center the eyes. Exhale and sweep the eyes all the way to the your right.

2. Inhale and move the eyes in a straight horizontal line to your left. Repeat 10 to 20 times. Close the eyes and rest.

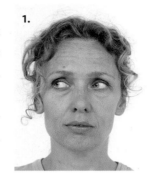
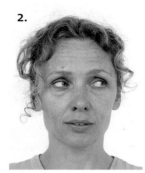

CIRCULAR MOVEMENTS

Sit in a comfortable position. Center the eyes. Imagine that there is a large clock face in front of you. Start by looking up toward twelve o'clock and move your eyes counterclockwise counting down every number on the clock from twelve to eleven and so on all the way around. Move the eyes slowly and smoothly like the second hand of a clock, touching every point around the periphery of the eyes. Repeat 4 to 10 times in both directions.

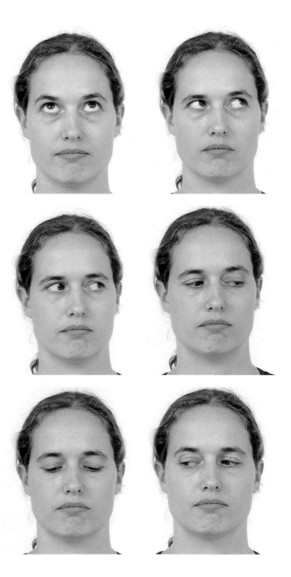

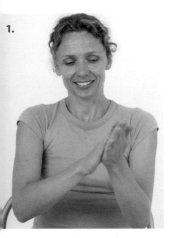

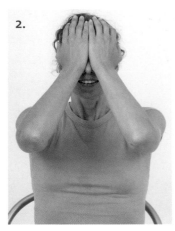

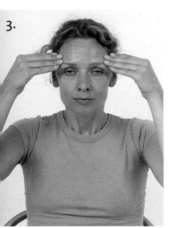

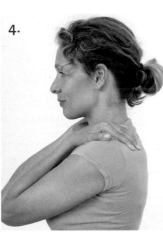

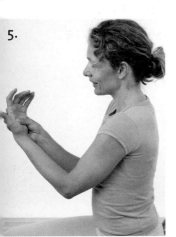

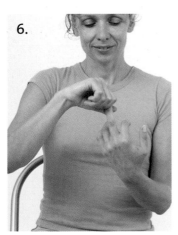

Post–eye exercise massage

1. Bring the hands into prayer position. Rub the palms together briskly until they feel hot.

2. Cup the palms over the eyes and bathe the eyes in the heat and darkness.

3. Massage the forehead and brow with the fingertips to release any tension around the eyes.

4. Then take the hands to the back of the neck and gently squeeze any tension from the neck and shoulders. Take hold of the opposite shoulder with each hand and continue massaging down the arms.

5. Gently squeeze and massage each palm with a circular thumb motion.

6. Softly pull the tip of each finger, to release tension through the hands and to loosen the joints.

Feet

The feet are often the most neglected and misused part of our anatomy. After decades of stuffing them into tight, ridiculously shaped shoes, it is no wonder that in later life the feet finally break down. Over the age of 40, as many as 80 percent of people have some type of foot problem, with women having four times as many problems as men.

The feet are an architectural wonder. The twenty-six bones in the feet are able to support and cushion the entire body weight, and to propel the body through space. The condition of the feet impacts the entire structure and alignment of the body. For instance, when we wear high-heeled shoes, the entire body weight is thrown forward onto the ball of the foot, causing the back to bend backward in order to compensate, resulting in numerous structural misalignments causing hip, knee, or back problems. Also the ankle is not properly supported and becomes weak and more prone to sprains and falls.

The beauty of yoga is that it is practiced in bare feet, giving a greater connection with the earth, which helps us to feel grounded. Numerous nerve endings in the feet correspond to each gland, organ, and part of the body, so massaging the feet relaxes and normalizes all the body's functions, restoring natural balance. Also, there are more sweat glands on the feet than anywhere else, so allowing air to circulate and the feet to breathe is a good practice.

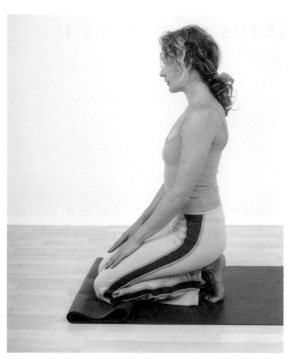

Foot exercises

The following yoga exercises help to stretch the feet and maintain flexibility in the toes.

Sitting toe strengthener

Come into a kneeling position. Stand up on both knees, with the knees hip-width apart and the toes tucked under. Sit back and place the buttocks on top of the heels. Hold for 20 seconds and release.

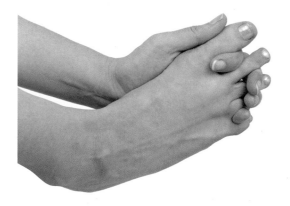

Toe stretching

Sit comfortably on a chair or the floor. Bend the right leg and place the right ankle on top of the left thigh, close to the left knee. Relax the right knee out to the side. Carefully insert the fingers between each toe, to create space between the toes. Hold for a few minutes. Repeat with the opposite foot.

Easing the Symptoms of Arthritis

Contrary to old beliefs, it is now recognized that arthritis sufferers need to remain active. When we are inactive, the muscles atrophy and it becomes increasingly harder to move, which triggers a negative downward spiral of inactivity, depression, and lethargy.

YOGA BENEFITS

Yoga has been shown to reduce the symptoms of arthritis, and is being used more and more for pain management. The movements help to increase joint mobility and to strengthen the muscles that support the body, which increases joint stability. Without exercise, the bones become brittle, leaving sufferers at greater risk of injury due to a fall. The yoga asanas strengthen the bones and restore agility and poise. The breathing and meditation practices also help to calm the nervous system, which helps people to cope with pain more effectively.

However, when beginning an exercise program it is important to respect pain. A stretching pain is good, but if sharp pain is experienced, always stop the exercise and rest. Never bounce in a pose as it can damage ligaments and tear muscles. Try to make the movements as fluid as possible following the natural line of motion of the joint. As an arthritis sufferer your range of motion may be limited, but in order to maintain joint mobility it is important to move each joint within its comfortable range.

Breathe steadily and evenly to send as much oxygen to the joints as possible, as this helps them perform at their best. Never hold your breath; we tend to hold the breath when concentrating, causing the muscles to tense and shorten, which may result in injury. Working in a heated room or having a hot bath or shower before practicing helps prepare the muscles and joints for the movements.

HOW TO PRACTICE

The following 35-minute program includes simple warm-up exercises that are gentle and restorative for arthritis sufferers. The exercises should be practiced regularly when pain and stiffness are at a minimum. For rheumatoid arthritis sufferers who tend to be stiff in the morning, an afternoon session is advisable: for osteoarthrhitis sufferers, who tend to get stiffer as the day progresses, a morning session is better. Getting started, especially when experiencing pain, is one of the most difficult hurdles. Begin slowly and rest between poses if necessary.

CAUTION

Yoga is not a substitute for allopathic or other medical therapies; rather, it is a complementary treatment to help alleviate the symptoms of disease. It is advisable to show this routine to your physician or physical therapist to determine the type and amount of exercise that it right for you.

EATING TO HELP ARTHRITIS

Recent findings link the edible nightshade family—potatoes, tomatoes, eggplant, pepper, and tobacco with joint pain and stiffness; removing them from the diet has helped many arthritis sufferers. Meat and wheat have also been found to be contributing factors. Vitamins A, C, and E are powerful antioxidants that protect the cartilage against the destructive effects of free radicals, so include plenty of foods containing these nutrients in your diet.

Asanas to help arthritis

Many of the following exercises can be practiced sitting on a firm chair.

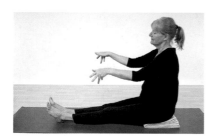
Head rolls (see p 49)

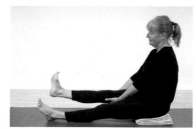
Shoulder circles (see p 50)

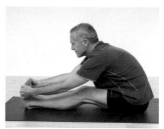
Elbow bends (see p 51)

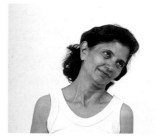
Wrist rotations (see p 51)

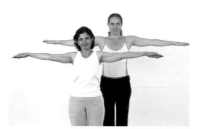
Ankle rolls (see p 51)

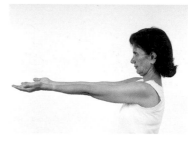
Forward bend (see p 81)

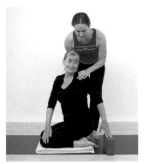

Side twist (see p 86)

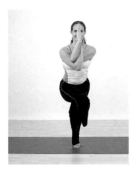

Eagle pose (see p 53)

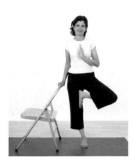

Tree pose with a chair
(see p 32)

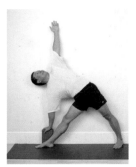

Triangle pose with block
(see p 34)

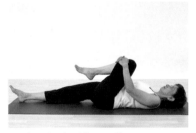

One knee to chest (see p 76)

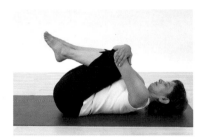

Both knees to chest (see p 76)

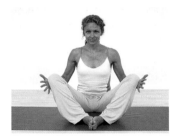

Cobbler pose (see p 84)

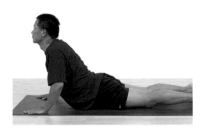

Cobra pose (see p 90)

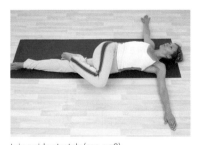

Lying side stretch (see p 78)

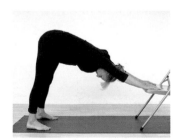

Downward dog with a chair (see p 32)

Getting Up and Down to the Floor

᧗

After a lifetime of sitting in chairs it becomes increasingly difficult to get down to the floor, which is necessary for many yoga postures. The action of getting up and down from the floor helps to keep the joints healthy and the body limber. For practitioners that are new to yoga or are suffering with arthritis, it is important to move slowly and safely to avoid injury.

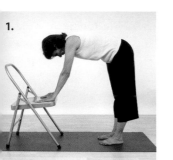

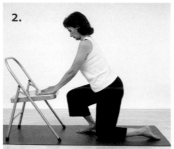

Getting down to the floor with a chair

1. Place a chair on the yoga mat, to prevent it from slipping, with the seat facing you. Stand in front of the chair about 2 feet (0.6 m) away. Bend forward and place your hands on the front of the chair.

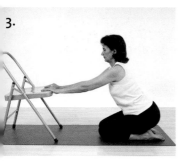

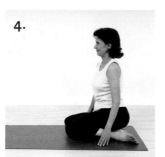

2. Step the right foot forward. Supporting your body weight with your arms, slowly bend the left knee down on to the floor.

3. Bend the right knee in line with the left and come to a kneeling position. Release the chair.

4. Lift the hips and take them to one side of the feet. Placing the hands down on the floor for additional support.

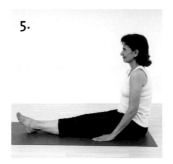

5. Swing the legs to one side, away from the hips. Extend the legs out in front with the feet together. To get up from the floor with the support of a chair, repeat the movements in the opposite direction.

Getting up from lying position

Lying flat on your back in *Savasana* is the final pose at the end of a yoga session.

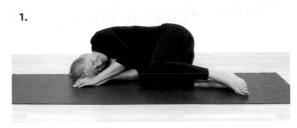

1. Bend the knees into the chest and roll to the right side. Rest for a few moments in a fetal position.

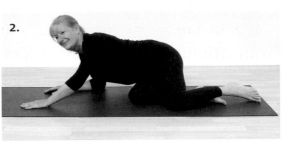

2. Place the left hand down onto the mat in front of the chest. Press into the left hand and begin to lift the torso up.

3. Come up onto your hands and knees and find your balance.

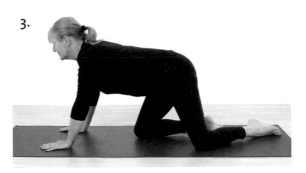

4. Bend the left knee and place the sole of the foot on the floor close to the hands.

5. Begin to shift the body weight into the hands and left foot and until you can step the right foot forward in line with the left. From a crouched position shift the body weight into both feet. Slowly come up to a standing position.

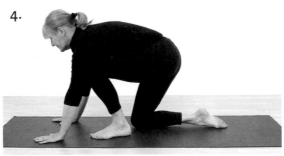

6. Stand in *tadasana* for a few moments to find your center.

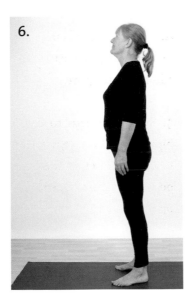

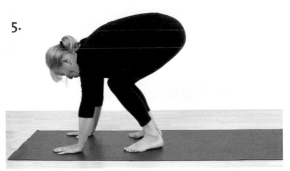

Helping the Symptoms of Heart Disease

Yoga is an amazing technique not only for working on the physical body but also on the deeper internal energy body. In the U.S. in 1990, a doctor named Dean Ornish first published his groundbreaking study showing that making lifestyle changes, including a healthy yoga diet, yoga exercise, meditation and positive thinking, can help heart disease. For one year, he treated a group of patients suffering with chronic heart disease with a program that included an hour a day of yoga, deep relaxation, meditation, and a vegetarian diet. By practicing yoga daily, his patients were able to reverse heart disease without the use of drugs and avoid bypass surgery.

WHAT ARE THE CONTRIBUTORY FACTORS

As we age various changes take place in the body, which may contribute to heart disease. Cholesterol, especially bad cholesterol (low-density lipoprotein, or LDL) increases; too much can cause clogged arteries and high blood pressure, which is another contributory factor in heart disease. Being overweight also puts us at higher risk, because the body has to work much harder to pump blood around the body.

However, the good news is that exercise reduces the level of bad cholesterol in the system and increases the good cholesterol. A healthy diet rich in vegetables, fruits, and grains is essential to prevent heart disease. Eating fewer saturated fats also helps prevent excessive weight gain.

HEALING STRESS

Stress is also a major contributor to heart disease. Deep relaxation during yoga induces a state of homeostasis, or balance, in the body, which helps to reduce stress. During breathing exercises, the heart accelerates on inhalation and slows on exhalation, so an extended exhalation helps to slow the heart and reduce blood pressure. When we do not breathe rhythmically, the heart is put under high stress.

PURIFYING THE HEART

According to yoga philosophy, another important dimension to the heart concerns the subtle energy body, the *nadis* or energy channels that form a network across the entire body (see page 17). At the heart center, the left and right channels are entwined particularly tightly around the central channel. The energy flowing in the inner channels, especially the left and right channels, is very connected to how we think. When we have strong negative emotions, the left and right channels swell and choke the central channel and block vital energy from flowing freely, thereby starving the heart. Yoga aims to purify negative emotions and reawaken the heart to experience the world with the freedom, innocence, and openness of a young child.

Asanas to help heart disease

The following *asanas* may help to relieve the symptoms of heart disease.

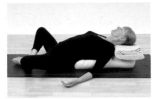

Cobbler pose with bolster (see p 28)

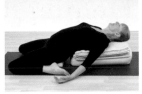

Hero pose with bolster (see p 29)

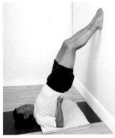

Shoulder stand with wall (see p 101)

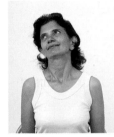

Head rolls (see p 49)

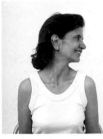

Head turns (see p 48)

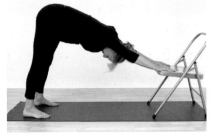

Downward dog with a chair (see p 32)

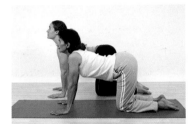

Cat pose (see p 52)

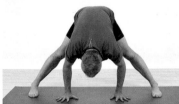

Extended leg pose (see p 68)

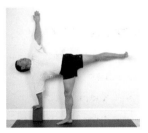

Half-moon pose (see p 43)

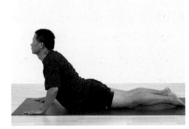

Cobra pose (see p 90)

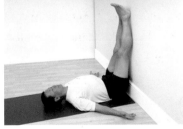

Legs up the wall (see p 42)

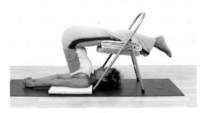

Plow pose with a chair (see p 33)

> ✳ **CAUTION** When suffering from heart disease it is important not to raise the arms over shoulder height.

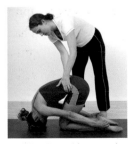

Baby head stand (see p 103)

To Restore the Body's Balance During Menopause

Menopause is part of the natural life cycle, which ushers in a new phase in a woman's existence. The change of life, when menstruation stops, is caused by a shift in hormone production. Perimenopause, or fluctuation in hormone production, starts a few years before menopause, between 45 and 55. This hormone flux can produce symptoms such as hot flashes, night sweats, insomnia, irritability, depression, and mood swings. These uncomfortable side-effects have created a general misconception of menopause as an age-related disease, which has prompted the medical community to produce a range of medications to help ease these effects.

HORMONE REPLACEMENT THERAPY

The main medication given to women over 45 is HRT, or hormone replacement therapy. After menopause, the ovaries produce less estrogen and progesterone, which the body requires to keep bones healthy and the body vital. Scientists believed that maintaining hormone levels at the old rate with a replacement hormone from mare's urine would remove the symptoms of menopause and actually slow the aging process. However, recent research has revealed that HRT may not be the miracle answer to eternal youth. HRT has been shown to increase the risk of cancer, particularly breast and endometrial cancer, and can cause blood clots. Increasing the level of progesterone, the sister hormone to estrogen, which helps to reduce the risk of cancer, has been found to increase the risk of heart disease, stroke, and cardiovascular problems.

MENOPAUSE AND LIFESTYLE

Each woman experiences menopause differently, and it is interesting to note that in other cultures where lifestyle follows a more natural rhythm, menopausal symptoms are practically nonexistent. Due to the many side-effects of replacement hormones, doctors now encourage women to pursue a healthy lifestyle, including a diet rich in fruit and vegetables, and exercises to strengthen the bones and heart. A number of natural plant supplements have been shown to prevent the symptoms of menopause including flaxseed oil, evening primrose oil, vitamin B6, vitamin E, and vitamin C. Eating soy is particularly good as it is high in a natural plant form of estrogen.

Menstrual cycles are governed by the endocrine system, especially the pituitary gland in the brain, which triggers the ovaries to produce estrogen and progesterone. Post-menopause, when the ovaries produce less estrogen, the adrenal glands take over and produce a form of estrogen called esterone, to maintain healthy bones. The practices of yoga are designed to stimulate the endocrine glands and keep them in good working order, thus helping to make the transitions of life smooth and symptom free. The more we are able to embrace the change of life the easier the transition. Many women find post-menopause to be a time of renewed vigor, energy, and freedom.

The following yoga exercises are recommended to ease the particular discomforts associated with menopause. Yoga aims to purify negative emotions and reawaken the heart to experience the world with the freedom, innocence, and openness of a young child.

For hot flashes and night sweats

Hot flashes are one of the most common symptoms of menopause where the body temperature rises causing the face, neck, and arms to blush. Supported forward bends are particularly recommended, as they are cooling and help calm the nervous system. Reclining poses like *supta baddhakonasana* and *supta virasana* help to open the chest, which improves breathing and also releases tension in the pelvis. Avoid eating spicy food, coffee, alcohol, and hot drinks as they create heat in the body.

To help anxiety and insomnia

During menopause, because of erratic hormone production, you can feel jittery and nervous, and suffer from anxiety and insomnia. The following poses help to calm the nervous system and restore harmony.

RESTORATIVE POSES

Restorative poses are particularly recommended for menopause, to help nourish and restore balance to the body. Restorative poses are postures that are practiced with the support of various props, which include a chair or wall, blocks, blankets, a belt or bolster, and are held for a few minutes. The props support the body in a posture, allowing you to relax more deeply into the pose. It is important to feel comfortable in a pose and, as each person's body has unique proportions, you will need to experiment to find the perfect height and placement of your prop.

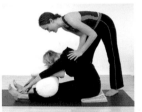
Forward bend with a bolster (see p 30)

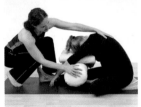
Head-to-knee pose with a bolster (see p 30)

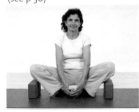
Cobbler pose with blocks (see p 35)

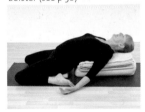
Hero pose with bolster (see p 29)

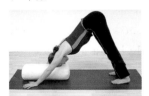
Downward dog with bolster (see p 29)

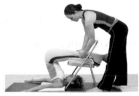
Plow pose with a chair (see p 33)

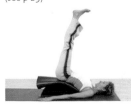
Half-shoulder stand with a back arch (see p 45)

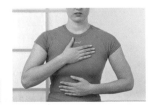
Full yogic breath (see p 22)

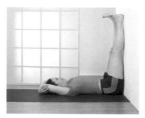
Legs up the wall (see p 42)

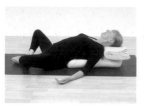
Bridge pose with a block (see p 35)

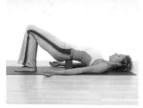
Cobbler pose with a bolster (see p 28)

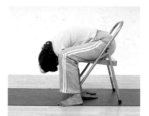
Forward bend with a chair (see p 31)

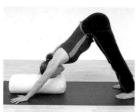
Downward dog with a bolster (see p 29)

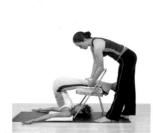
Plow pose with a chair (see p 33)

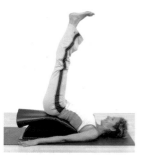
Half-shoulder stand with a back arch (see p 45) or Shoulder stand with a blanket (see p 36)

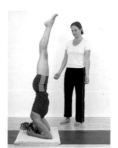
Headstand (see p 104)

To relieve fatigue

The internal changes during menopause can often result in a general malaise. The following *asanas* are good for overcoming fatigue.

Legs up the wall, or *vaparita karani,* can help you feel grounded if you're suffering from a bout of indecision. It is one of the most healing of the yoga poses, reducing the heart rate and promoting deep relaxation. It is also good for mild hypertension.

Gentle, supported back-bends help to stimulate the adrenal glands and lift the spirits, try the following exercises for increased vitality.

Muddled thoughts

The mind often gets cloudy and muddled during menopause, resulting in indecisiveness. To help improve the functioning of the mind inversions are highly recommended along with deep breathing to send oxygen and nutrients to the brain, though it is not recommended to practice inversions during menstruation.

> **HERBS FOR HORMONE BALANCE**
> The following herbs help balance progesterone/estrogen levels: alfalfa, Chinese ginseng, licorice root, raspberry leaves and fennel.

OSTEOPOROSIS

One of the most chronic diseases that can be a by-product of post-menopause is osteoporosis. Brittle bones, or reduced bone density due to reduced levels of progesterone and estrogen, characterizes osteoporosis. In the US, 10 million people suffer from osteoporosis, 80 percent of whom are post-menopausal women. Osteoporosis can progress painlessly until a bone breaks. The areas of the body that are most susceptible are the hip, spine, and wrists. A hip fracture almost always requires hospitalization and major surgery. Spinal fractures can result in a loss of height, severe back pain, and deformity.

However, osteoporosis in not an inevitable result of menopause. Recommended prevention for osteoporosis focuses on a healthy diet and proper exercise. A healthy balanced diet is one rich in nutrients. For people suffering from osteoporosis, the intake of calcium from dairy products, especially yogurt and cheese, is recommended, along with collard greens and broccoli. Vitamin D is another essential nutrient that increases calcium absorption. It can be best absorbed by sitting in the sun for 15 minutes a day. Fish oil is another good source of Vitamin D. Cutting out cigarettes and alcohol is also advisable as both activities increase the likelihood of brittle bones, while salt leeches calcium from the bones so is also best avoided.

Exercise, especially weight-bearing exercises, are essential in the prevention of osteoporosis. When we place weight on a particular limb, the muscles send a message to the bone causing it to thicken and become strong. Another advantage of regular exercise is that the muscles get firmer, which act as a shock absorber and can cushion a fall, preventing bone damage.

Yoga is a great weight-bearing form of exercise, as the poses redistribute the weight to various parts of the body in a safe and gentle way, allowing the body to build up more strength over time. Balancing poses and inversions are especially bone-strengthening exercises, placing the body weight on one leg, or the head or hands, for example. They also improve overall balance and agility in later life. The ability to balance is one of the last motor-neuron skills we learn as children and one of the first to go in later life, so it is important to prolong the ability through regular practice.

Stress is also a contributing factor to osteoporosis, as it creates acidity in the blood that contributes to bone depletion. The breathing techniques, meditation, and deep relaxation are useful in reducing stress and making the blood more alkaline, which is better for internal health.

GLOSSARY

Amma Accumulated toxins, undigested food, and waste material in the body.

Anandamaya Kosha The field of limitless potential.

Annamaya Kosha The physical body.

Asana Yoga posture. Literally, "steady, comfortable pose."

Chakras Energy centers. Literally, "wheels."

Dandasana Staff pose; the neutral sitting pose for all forward bends.

Kapalabhati breathing Rapid diaphragmatic breathing that removes impurities from the body.

Manomaya Kosha The mind body.

Nadis Energy channels that form a network across our entire bodies; the channels radiating energy from the chakras.

Prana Energy; life force. Referred to as *chi* by the Chinese.

Pranamaya Kosha The energy body.

Pranayama Breathing exercises that rhythmically control the breath. Literally, "expansion of the life force."

Savasana Relaxation on the back. Gives the body time to absorb the full benefits of the practice.

Surya Namaskar Sun salutation; a dynamic series of fourteen asanas linked together with the breath.

Tadasana Primary standing pose that teaches realignment and balance.

Ujjai breathing Breathing technique whereby you gently contract the glottis to produce a soft snoring sound at the back of the throat.

Vijnanamaya Kosha Awareness.

Yoga Union. To yoke or to join; to attach the mind to one object and to penetrate its essential nature.

Yoga Nidra Deep relaxation, or "yoga sleep." Allows the benefits of the asanas to be assimilated.

INDEX

Exercice 6 •••••••••••••••••

Carnet de notes

1 Trouvez dans le texte les mots de liaison et les phrases qui suivent et notez-les. Vous pourrez ensuite les réutiliser dans vos rédactions ou dans vos discussions en français:

dû à	due to
afin de	in order to, so as to
selon	according to
tout en (+ verbe + ant)	while (doing something)
bien que	although
ainsi	thus

2 Parcourez une dernière fois le texte et notez au moins 8 autres mots ou expressions que vous allez apprendre. N'oubliez pas de les noter en contexte.

Exercice 7 •••••••••••••••

Passage à l'écrit

Reprenez les notes que vous avez prises pour l'exercice 2, ainsi que le corrigé de cet exercice. A l'aide de ces notes écrivez un court article sur les recherches sur les risques de leucémie, les groupes à risque et les mesures qui vont être prises suite au débat. Essayez de réutiliser le vocabulaire que vous avez appris ainsi que les mots de liaison qui conviennent.

Ecrivez un maximum de 200 mots.

Exercice 3 •••••••••••••••

Utilisation de la construction '(se) faire + verbe à l'infinitif'(+à)'

Traduisez les phrases suivantes en français en vous servant de la construction '(se) faire + verbe à l'infinitif':

1 We're going to have a house built in Brittany.
2 He's going to get the car fixed tomorrow.
3 The film made me cry.
4 If we go out this evening the au pair will feed the children.
5 She had a delicious meal made.

Exercice 4 •••••••••••••••••••••••••••••••••••••••

Elargissement du vocabulaire

Relisez le texte et ensuite à l'aide de votre dictionnaire remplissez les cases ci-dessous avec d'autres mots de la même famille que celui qui vous est donné en caractères gras. (Suivez l'exemple du mot 'publier'). Attention, vous ne pourrez pas remplir toutes les cases dans la colonne 'adverbes'.

verbes	noms	adjectifs / participes	adverbes
publier	**la publication** **la publicité**	**publicitaire**	
		médical	
	le débat		
		paru	
		convaincant	
	la consommation		
		pêché	
			localement
fréquenter			
accroître			
		comparable	
		accueilli	
	le prélèvement		
vérifier			
		étayé	

Le Nucléaire et la Santé

Exercice 5 ••

Mots croisés

Remplissez ce mots croisés à l'aide des phrases ci-dessous. Les mots manquant dans les phrases marquées d'un * sont tirés de l'exercice 4 et les autres sont tirés du texte lui-même.

horizontalement

1   le contraire de 's'attrister' (2,7)

2   * Il faut _____ (8) de nouveau le problème des risques de leucémie dus au nucléaire.

3   L'étude a été _____ (5) par le professeur Viel

4   un synonyme de 'au bout de' (1, 1, 9, 2)

5   Ceux qui _____ (10) régulièrement des crustacés et des poissons pêchés localement courent un risque.

6   le contraire de 'défendu' (8)

7   un synonyme du 'cancer des cellules du sang' (8)

8   * Je me fais du souci pour mon fils. Il sort avec des gens qui ne sont pas très _____ (13)

verticalement

1   un synonyme de 'près de' (1, 9, 2)

2   le contraire de 'décroître' (9)

3   Ceux qui _____ (11) les plages de La Hague courent un risque accru de leucémie.

4   * Ses chaussures la font _____ (8) plus grande.

5   Il faut prêter attention à cette étude sérieuse et très _____ (6) du professeur Viel.

6   un synonyme de 'magazine' (5)

Observations linguistiques

The prefix 're–'

In the text there are four examples of words beginning with the prefix 're-':

relancer (para 1)

retraitement (para 3)

rejeter (para 10)

ressortir (para 6)

As in English the prefix 're-' in French usually implies doing something again, or starting something again. Look at how the phrases containing these prefixes may be translated in English. You will see that the first two sentences are more straightforward than the last ones, which do not really carry the meaning of doing or starting something again in either the French or the English.

1)   'une étude ... **re**lance le débat'
     *a study ... has **re**vived the debate*

2)   'près du vaste complexe de **re**traitement de combustibles nucléaires usés'
     *near the huge nuclear fuel **re**processing plant*

3)   'l'usine de La Hague est autorisée à **re**jeter 800 fois plus de radionucléides en mer que la plus grande centrale nucléaire française, celle de Gravelines.'
     *the plant at La Hague is allowed to **dis**charge 800 times more radionuclides into the sea than Gravelines, the largest French nuclear power station.*

4)   'plusieurs recherches menées en Grande Bretagne ... avaient fait **res**sortir des risques de leucémie infantile accrus.'
     several studies carried out in Great Britain ... had brought out the increased risk of infantile leukaemia
     Note that in this case an extra 's' is added to the prefix to ensure that the 's' in 'sortir' is not pronounced as a 'z'. (other examples of this are 'ressouder', 'ressembler', 'resservir').

Here are examples of some other words from the text from which we could form related words by using the prefix 're-':

word in text	related word beginnng with 're-'	English translation
publier	republier	to republish
annoncer	réannoncer	to announce again
vérifier	revérifier	to verify again
établir	rétablir	to re-establish
pêcher	repêcher	to fish out, to recover (body)
tomber malade	retomber malade	to fall ill again
poser (une question)	reposer (une question)	to ask (a question) again
une évaluation	une réévaluation	a re-evaluation

Note that, as in the case of 'réannoncer' and 'réévaluation', where the prefix 're-' is followed by a vowel, it becomes 'ré-'.

JENNY OLLERENSHAW © 1998, 2002

JENNY OLLERENSHAW © 1998, 2002

Corrigés et Explications

Exercice 1 •

mots-clés	définitions
la leucémie	cancer des cellules du sang
épidémiologique	relatif à l'étude des différents facteurs qui interviennent dans l'apparition des maladies
à proximité de	près de
engager	commencer
convaincant	décisif
infantile	qui touche les petits enfants
le retraitement de combustibles nucléaires usés	opération qui permet de récupérer les éléments fissiles et fertiles en les séparant des produits de fission fortement radioactifs
à l'extrémité de	au bout de
une association	relation
les crustacés	fruits de mer tels que les crabes, les crevettes, les langoustes
fréquenter	aller souvent dans un lieu
accroître	augmenter
la prudence	précaution
le prélèvement	action de prendre une certaine portion sur une masse
étayé	soutenu par des exemples
l'unanimité	conformité d'opinion entre tous les membres d'un groupe

4

Exercice 2 • • • • • • • • • • • • • •

le sujet de débat

le risque plus grand de leucémies à proximité des grandes installations nucléaires

les groupes à risque

- Les enfants qui habitent près des grandes installations nucléaires (en France, en particulier les enfants qui habitent à proximité du complexe de retraitement de combustibles nucléaires usés de la COGEMA à la Hague et, en Grande Bretagne, ceux qui habitent près de Sellafield et Dounreay).

- Les personnes qui consomment au moins une fois par semaine des poissons et crustacés pêchés localement.

- les personnes qui fréquentent les plages

les résultats des recherches menées en France et en Grande Bretagne

Les chercheurs dans les deux pays s'accordent pour dire que les groupes ci-dessus courent un plus grand risque de leucémie. Selon l'étude française les risques sont trois fois plus importants à la Hague qu'ailleurs.

la réaction des autorités françaises

- Les autorités françaises ont accueilli l'étude avec prudence.

- l'INSERM remet en question l'interprétation des résultats

- la CRII-RAD (Commission de Recherche et d'Information Indépendante sur la Radioactivité) ne s'est pas prononcée sur l'étude mais se dit heureuse 'qu'une étude épidémiologique indépendante ait pu être publiée.'

les mesures qui vont être prises suite au débat

- Le ministre de l'Environnement et le secretaire d'état à la Santé vont lancer une nouvelle 'étude épidémiologique complète' pour vérifier l'incidence des cas de leucémie dans plusieurs cantons de la Manche

- Les autorités françaises ont annoncé un renforcement des études épidémiologiques par l'INSERM près de la Hague

- Madame Lepage, le ministre de l'Environnement, a demandé une évaluation de l'étude du professeur Viel et elle va faire pratiquer des prélèvements d'eau et de coquillages en mer, pour vérifier qu'il n'y a pas de concentration de radioactivité "anormale"

Exercice 3 • • • • • • • • • • • • • •

1) On va **se faire construire** une maison en Bretagne. *(in this case the house will be built for <u>them</u> to live in)*

On va **faire construire** une maison en Bretagne. *(in this case the house could be built either for themselves or for <u>someone else</u> to live in)*

2) Il va **faire réparer** la voiture demain.

3) Le film m'a **fait pleurer**.

4) Si nous sortons/on sort ce soir la jeune fille au pair **fera manger/dîner** les enfants.

5) Elle a **fait préparer** un repas délicieux.

JENNY OLLERENSHAW © 1998, 2002

4

Corrigés et Explications

Exercice 4 •

verbes	noms	adjectifs/ participes	adverbes
publier	la publication la publicité	publicitaire	
médicaliser	la médecine le médecin la médication le médicament la médicalisation	médical médicamenteux médicinal	médicalement
débattre	le débat	débattu	
paraître	le paraître la parution	paru	apparemment
convaincre se convaincre	la conviction	convaincant convaincu	
consommer	la consommation le consommateur	consommable consommé	
pêcher	la pêche la pêcherie le pêcheur	pêché	
localiser	le local la localisation	local localisable	localement
fréquenter se fréquenter	la fréquentation	fréquentable fréquenté	
accroître	l'accroissement	accru	
comparer	la comparaison	comparable comparatif comparé	comparativement
accueillir	l'accueil	accueilli accueillant	
prélever	le prélèvement		
vérifier	la vérification le vérificateur	vérifiable	
étayer	l'étayage	étayé	

41

4

Exercice 5 ....

Corrigés et Explications

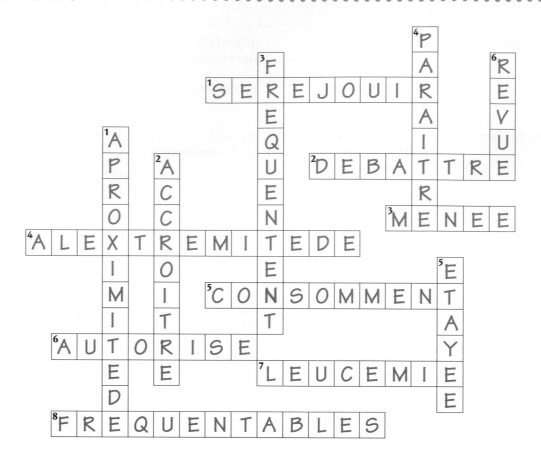

JENNY OLLERENSHAW © 1998, 2002

5   L'Euthanasie

Esquisse d'une philosophie de l'ADMD

Réflexions d'un adhérent

Les adversaires de l'ADMD, mal informés ou de mauvaise foi, essaient de nous faire passer pour des maniaques atteints d'un morbide vertige de mort, pour des "pousse au suicide". Ne craignons pas d'opposer à cette caricature la philosophie qui inspire les adhérents de l'ADMD. Cette philosophie repose essentiellement sur l'amour de la vie, un amour de la vie lucide, qui n'empêche pas la conscience et l'acceptation de notre condition d'êtres mortels. Elle s'accompagne en outre d'une grande exigence de liberté.

AMOUR DE LA VIE

Comme tous les êtres humains, nous aimons la vie et la souhaitons aussi longue que possible. Nous déplorons la mort, volontaire ou non, des êtres jeunes et valides. Loin de pousser au suicide, les responsables de l'ADMD ont plus d'une fois redonné des raisons de vivre à ceux qui croyaient n'en plus avoir.

Mais c'est précisément parce que nous aimons la vie que nous voulons mourir vivants, que nous voulons préserver jusqu'au bout la qualité et la dignité d'une vie que nous refusons de confondre avec les dérisoires et pitoyables prolongations qu'on voudrait nous imposer au nom de la morale et de la médecine!

De plus, aimer la vie, ce n'est pas seulement s'accrocher à sa propre existence, c'est aussi penser à la vie des autres. Nous ne pouvons supporter l'idée que, pour nous conserver une caricature de vie dont nous ne voulons plus, soient imposées aux nôtres une épreuve intolérable et à la société une charge insupportable.

L'amour de la vie ne s'accommode ni de la dégradation ni de l'égoïsme.

ACCEPTATION DE LA MORT

La mort est le grand scandale de la condition humaine, source de révolte et d'angoisse.

Dans leur lutte pour prolonger la vie, les hommes ont remporté des succès. Mais l'homme est toujours mortel.

Un adhérent de l'ADMD accepte cette réalité. Après s'être battu pour conserver une vie digne, quand la lutte est devenue sans espoir, maîtrisant son angoisse, il veut regarder la mort en face et choisir son heure. Il refuse les lentes agonies, les souffrances terminales, la déchéance physique et mentale.

On comprend difficilement que cette attitude - la seule compatible avec la dignité de l'homme - rencontre une si grande incompréhension, une opposition souvent hargneuse, parfois malhonnête. Trop de contemporains refusent la mort et pensent lui échapper en prolongeant par tous les moyens une vie dégradée dont elle s'est déjà emparée.

EXIGENCE DE LIBERTÉ

Dans nos sociétés libérales et libérées, on se plaît à réclamer toutes les libertés, fût-ce aux dépens des autres et au détriment de la discipline et de la cohésion sociales.

Or, on nous refuse une liberté fondamentale, qui ne lèse personne et ne nuit pas à la société: celle de choisir les conditions et l'heure de notre mort. Liberté pour nous-mêmes, quand nous jugeons que notre vie est dégradée au point de devenir intolérable, d'obtenir qu'on ne la prolonge pas et même qu'éventuellement on nous aide à l'abréger de façon digne. Liberté pour ceux qui nous entourent de pouvoir, dans ce cas, nous apporter leur aide, sans être considérés comme des meurtriers.

Mais, en même temps, nous demandons la liberté de vivre et de lutter en bénéficiant de tous les moyens qui abolissent la douleur et corrigent les handicaps. Et ceux qui veulent vivre le plus longtemps possible, quel que soit leur état, ont évidemment droit à toutes les aides nécessaires.

Dans ce drame de la vie et de la mort, au-delà des préjugés et des principes fallacieux, l'important est de respecter la liberté de chacun, liberté qui, tempérée par la conscience exigeante de nos responsabilités, constitue, avec l'amour de la vie et l'acceptation de la mort, les fondements de la sagesse humaine.

L'Association pour le Droit de Mourir dans la Dignité.

5

L'Euthanasie

Exercice 1 • • • • • • • • • • • • • • • • •

Compréhension des mots–clés

Dans ce dépliant publié par *l'Association pour le Droit de Mourir dans la Dignité* certains mots ont un sens positif et d'autres, un sens négatif. Avant de lire le dépliant classez donc ces mots, selon leur sens, dans la colonne 'sens positif' ou 'sens négatif'. S'il y a des mots que vous ne connaissez pas essayez de deviner à quelle colonne ils vont appartenir avant de chercher leur sens dans le dictionnaire. Cet exercice va vous préparer pour la lecture du texte.

Exemple:

sens positif	sens négatif
l'amour de la vie	déplorer

déplorer	sans espoir
apporter une aide	la mauvaise foi
dérisoire	bénéficier de
hargneux	maniaque
l'amour de la vie	la dégradation
malhonnête	digne
pitoyable	préserver
léser	morbide
l'épreuve	l'égoïsme
nuire à	imposer
la dignité	l'angoisse
la qualité	la sagesse
intolérable	les lentes agonies
les préjugés	la caricature
la charge	vivant
fallacieux	les souffrances
insupportable	la déchéance
la liberté	terminales

Exercice 2 • • • • • • • • • • • • • • •

Compréhension des mots–clés

1 Lisez maintenant le texte et trouvez les expressions/les phrases en français qui correspondent à ces expressions/phrases en anglais:

   a Opponents of l'ADMD ... try to make us out to be cranks

   b This philosophy is essentially based on a love of life ...

   c Far from encouraging people to commit suicide

   d clinging onto one's own existence

   e We can't stand the idea that ...

   f ... Man has been successful

   g After having fought to retain a dignified life

   h ... (s)he wants to look death in the face and choose his/her hour

   i we enjoy demanding every freedom, even if it is at the expense of others

   j And those who want to live as long as possible, whatever their condition

2 Regardez bien le corrigé et apprenez les expressions en caractères gras. Vous en aurez besoin pour l'exercice 4.

Exercice 3 • • • • • • • • • • • • • •

Compréhension du texte

Répondez aux questions suivantes en anglais. L'ordre des questions suit l'ordre du texte.

1 According to the text how do ADMD's opponents caricature them?

2 What is the philosophy that inspires members of the ADMD?

3 How does the ADMD refute the allegation that they push people into committing suicide?

4 According to the ADMD's philosophy is the quality of a person's life important? What do they say about it?

5 In what way does this philosophy encompass the feelings and position of people other than the dying person?

6 According to the ADMD what is the reality of death?

7 When death is near what is the attitude of the ADMD's members?

8 How do some people outside the organisation react to this attitude?

9 Which freedom do they claim that society refuses us?

10 In the eyes of the ADMD what forms the foundations of human wisdom?

Exercice 4 • • • • • • • • • • • • • •

Réutilisation du vocabulaire et des structures

Cet exercice va vous permettre de réutiliser le vocabulaire et les structures que vous avez vus dans le texte. Avant de le faire regardez de nouveau le corrigé de l'exercice 2. Ensuite traduisez les phrases suivantes en français:

1 The success of the project is based on the efficiency of the workers.

JENNY OLLERENSHAW © 1998, 2002

2 You have to look danger in the face before making your first parachute jump.

3 She can't stand her father's selfishness.

4 Far from harming society this project will bring help to the poorest people in the capital.

5 In spite of his physical decline he is clinging to life.

6 Whatever the financial difficulties of the hospitals, they do not have the right to economise at the expense of the patients.

7 My doctor is trying to make me out to be an invalid!

8 The important thing is not to impose unbearable burdens on society.

9 After having trained for five years he was successful in the European and World Championships.

10 Many doctors try desperately to prolong patients' lives no matter what their mental and physical state is.

Exercice 5 • • • • • • • • • • • • • • •

Compréhension du texte

D'après vous lesquelles des phrases suivantes auraient pu être prononcées par un adhérent de l'ADMD?

1 Il n'est pas toujours bon de prolonger la vie d'un patient.

2 Nous déplorons l'euthanasie.

3 Ceux qui aident les gens à abréger leur vie sont des meurtriers.

4 Si on aime la vie on ne peut pas accepter notre condition d'êtres mortels.

5 Il est préférable de mourir plutôt que de poursuivre une vie qui n'est plus digne.

6 Si on aime la vie on pense aussi à la souffrance de ses proches quand on est gravement malade.

7 Si un jeune valide voulait abréger sa vie nous soutiendrions son choix.

8 Si j'adhère à l'ADMD cela veut dire que je ne veux pas de déchéance physique et mentale à la fin de ma vie.

9 Je veux vivre le plus longtemps possible, quel que soit mon état.

10 Chacun devrait pouvoir choisir d'abréger ou de prolonger sa vie s'il souffre d'une maladie en phase terminale.

11 Les adhérents de l'ADMD sont obsédés par la mort.

12 Si on aime la vie on fait tout pour ne pas mourir.

Exercice 6 •

Carnet de notes

1 Trouvez dans le texte les mots de liaison et les phrases qui suivent et notez-les. Vous pourrez ensuite les réutiliser dans vos rédactions ou dans vos discussions en français:

2 Parcourez une dernière fois le texte et notez au moins 8 autres mots ou expressions. N'oubliez pas de les noter en contexte.

en outre	in addition
loin de (+ infinitif)	far from (+ verb + ing)
précisément	precisely
de plus	furthermore
aux dépens de	at the expense of
or	and yet
quel que soit ...	whatever ... may be
au-delà de	beyond
l'important est de	the important thing is to
au détriment de	to the detriment of
tempéré par	tempered by

Exercice 7 •

Passage à l'écrit

Ecrivez une rédaction de 200 à 250 mots dans laquelle vous expliquerez pourquoi vous êtes pour ou contre l'euthanasie. Essayez de réutiliser les expressions et le vocabulaire que vous avez vus dans le texte.

Corrigés et Explications

Exercice 1 ● ● ● ● ● ● ● ● ● ● ● ● ● ●

sens positif	sens négatif
l'amour de la vie	déplorer
la dignité	dérisoire
bénéficier de	pitoyable
préserver	l'épreuve
apporter une aide	intolérable
vivant	la charge
la qualité	insupportable
la liberté	sans espoir
digne	intolérable
la sagesse	la dégradation
	l'égoïsme
	l'angoisse
	les lentes agonies
	la déchéance
	hargneux
	malhonnête
	léser
	nuire à
	les préjugés
	fallacieux
	la mauvaise foi
	maniaque
	morbide
	imposer
	la caricature
	les souffrances terminales

Exercice 2 ● ● ● ● ● ● ● ● ● ● ● ● ● ●

1 Opponents of l'ADMD ... try **to make us out to be** cranks

Les adversaires de l'ADMD ... essaient de **nous faire passer pour** des maniaques

2 This philosophy is essentially **based on** a love of life ...

Cette philosophie **repose** esentiellement **sur** l'amour de la vie ...

3 **Far from** encouraging people to commit suicide

loin de pousser au suicide

4 **clinging onto** one's own existence

s'accrocher à sa propre existence

5 **We can't stand** the idea that ...

Nous ne pouvons supporter l'idée que ... *Here the 'pas' of the negative has been omitted for reasons of style*

6 ... Man **has been successful**

... les hommes **ont remporté des succès**

7 **After having fought** to retain a dignified life

Après s'être battu pour conserver une vie digne

You probably remember the expression 'après avoir + past participle' meaning 'after having + past participle'. Don't forget that if the verb is a reflexive one, or one of the list that always takes the auxilliary 'être' in the perfect tense, then you must say 'après (s')être + past participle'

8 ... (s)he wants **to look death in the face** and choose his/her hour

... il veut **regarder la mort en face** et choisir son heure

Note that where in English we might choose to use he/she, French keeps to the rule of using the masculine form to represent both sexes.

9 **we enjoy demanding** every freedom, even if it is **at the expense of** others

on se plaît à réclamer toutes les libertés, fût-ce **aux dépens des** autres

JENNY OLLERENSHAW © 1998, 2002

Note that there is a typing error in the text: 'fut-ce' should actually be 'fût-ce' since it is a subjunctive.

10 And those who want to live as long as possible, **whatever** their condition

Et ceux qui veulent vivre le plus longtemps possible, **quel que soit** leur état

Exercice 3 ● ● ● ● ● ● ● ● ● ● ● ● ● ● ● ● ●

1 They think that they are crazy people with a morbid obsession with death who push people into committing suicide.

2 Their philosophy is essentially based on a love of life, a clear-sighted love of life which does not preclude an awareness and acceptance of our mortality. It goes hand-in-hand with a strong demand for freedom.

3 They say that far from doing this they have, on more than one occasion, given a reason to live to those who thought that there was no more reason to live.

4 Yes, they think it is of vital importance. They believe that it is vital to maintain the quality and dignity of one's life to the end. They say that this should not be confused with the pathetic and pitiful lenthening of life that medicine and morality want to impose on us.

5 They feel that if one loves life it does not mean one should cling to one's own existence, but that one should also think of the life of others. They can't stand the thought that, in order to preserve a caricature of life that they don't even want any more, their loved ones should be subjected to an intolerable ordeal, and that society should bear a dreadful burden.

6 Death is the great scandal of the human condition. It is a source of revolt and anguish. Although great progress has been made in prolonging life, Man is still mortal.

7 If the fight for a dignified life is hopeless, the ADMD member tries to control his anxiety, looks death in the face and chooses his time of death. He refuses to suffer slow agonies, terminal suffering and physical and mental decline. ADMD members see such an attitude as the only one compatible with Man's dignity.

8 ADMD members say that it meets with a great lack of understanding and an opposition which is often aggressive and sometimes dishonest.

9 That of choosing the conditions and the time of our death. The freedom for us to decide as individuals, when we consider that our life has deteriorated to the point of being intolerable, that we no longer wish our life to be prolonged and even possibly that we be helped to end it in a dignified manner. The freedom for those around us to be able, under these circumstances, to help us without being thought of as murderers.

10 The ADMD believes that the freedom of everyone has to be respected. This freedom, tempered by the demanding awareness of our responsibilities, and hand-in-hand with the love of life and the acceptance of death, forms the foundations of human wisdom.

Exercice 4 ● ● ● ● ● ● ● ● ● ● ● ● ● ● ● ● ●

1 La réussite du projet repose sur l'efficacité des travailleurs.

2 Il faut regarder le danger en face avant de faire son premier saut en parachute / Vous devez regarder le danger en face avant de faire votre premier saut en parachute.

3 Elle ne peut (pas) supporter l'égoïsme de son père.

Note that for stylistic reasons the 'pas' can be omitted. This is often the case when the verbs 'pouvoir', 'cesser' and 'oser' are negated.

4 Loin de nuire à la société ce projet apportera une aide aux plus pauvres de la capitale.

5 Malgré sa déchéance physique il s'accroche à la vie.

6 Quelles que soient les difficultés financières des hôpitaux, ils n'ont pas le droit d'économiser aux dépens des patients.

7 Mon médecin essaie de me faire passer pour un(e) invalide!

8 L'important est de ne pas imposer de charges insupportables à la société.

9 Après s'être entraîné pendant cinq ans il a remporté des succès dans les championnats européen et mondial.

Did you remember to use the auxilliary 'être' with this reflexive verb?

10 Beaucoup de médecins s'acharnent à prolonger la vie des patients, quel que soit leur état mental et physique.

5

Corrigés et Explications

Exercice 5 ● ● ● ● ● ● ● ● ● ● ● ● ● ● ●

We have chosen the following sentences. If you are unsure as to why they were chosen use the short explanation given in English to find the relevant passage in the text.

1 Il n'est pas toujours bon de prolonger la vie d'un patient.

(Amour de la vie) *They believe that the **quality** of a patient's life is of great importance. If the patient no longer has a good quality of life then they believe that there is no point in prolonging the life.*

5 Il est préférable de mourir plutôt que de poursuivre une vie qui n'est plus digne.

The reason is the same as for number 1.

6 Si on aime la vie on pense aussi à la souffrance de ses proches quand on est gravement malade.

(Amour de la vie) *They believe that one should think about the burden that one represents to others when termianally ill.*

8 Si j'adhère à l'ADMD cela veut dire que je ne veux pas de déchéance physique et mentale à la fin de ma vie.

(Acceptation de la mort) *They refuse slow agonies, terminal suffering and physical and mental decline.*

10 Chacun devrait pouvoir choisir d'abréger ou de prolonger sa vie s'il souffre d'une maladie en phase terminale.

(Exigence de liberté) *They do not want to impose euthanasia on anyone, but believe that everyone should have the right to decide whether they want their life to be prolonged or not.*

The following are unlikely to have been said by an ADMD member for the reasons given:

2 Nous déplorons l'euthanasie.

This is exactly what they are advocating throughout the text.

3 Ceux qui aident les gens à abréger leur vie sont des meurtriers.

(Exigence de liberté) *This is the view that prevails in society as a whole, and it is what they want to change.*

4 Si on aime la vie on ne peut pas accepter notre condition d'êtres mortels.

(Acceptation de la mort) *Man is still mortal, and ADMD members accept this reality.*

7 Si un jeune valide voulait abréger sa vie nous soutiendrions son choix.

(Amour de la vie) *They are totally against the death of young, healthy people, whether they choose to die or not.*

9 Je veux vivre le plus longtemps possible quel que soit mon état.

In several places the text makes it clear that to ADMD members life is only worth living if it is dignified and they still have a reasonable quality of life.

11 Les adhérents de l'ADMD sont obsédés par la mort.

(Introduction) *They say that outsiders often mistake them for being obsessed by death, but that this is not true.*

12 Si on aime la vie on fait tout pour ne pas mourir.

See number 9.

JENNY OLLERENSHAW © 1998, 2002

6 La Pollution

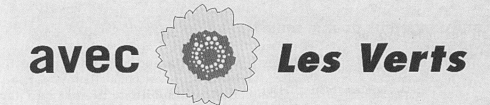

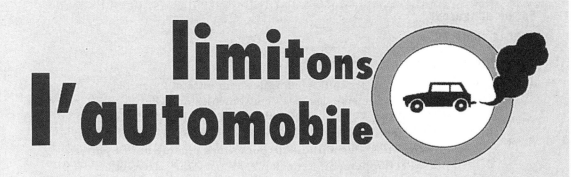

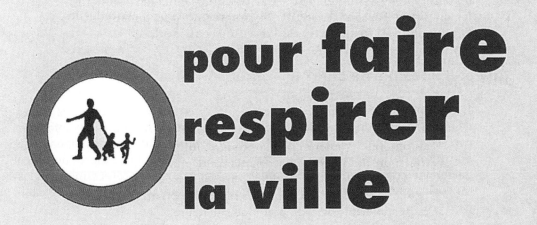

ADHÉREZ AUX VERTS : 107 avenue Parmentier - 75011 Paris - minitel 36.14 LES VERTS

6

La Pollution

L'air que nous respirons est-il pollué?

Incontestablement, l'air des villes est de plus en plus pollué. La pollution due aux industries a fortement diminué, mais la pollution due à l'automobile ne cesse d'augmenter: l'ozone, les oxydes d'azote, les oxydes de carbone et les particules fines prolifèrent.

Est-il dangereux pour la santé?

Oui. Toutes les études médicales le montrent. Quand la pollution augmente, les crises d'asthme, les maladies respiratoires, les conjonctivites, les maux de têtes et la mortalité augmentent. **L'automobile ne tue pas que par les accidents, elle tue aussi des milliers de personnes chaque année par ses pots d'échappement.** Les enfants, les personnes âgées et les asthmatiques sont les principales victimes, mais tout le monde est touché. De plus, le diesel introduit une pollution particulièrement dangereuse: il émet des particules fines qui s'accumulent dans les poumons, provoquant des maladies respiratoires et cardio-vasculaires, et qui seraient cancérigènes.

Comment en est-on arrivé là?

Depuis 30 ans la politique des transports se limite au "tout-automobile": autoroutes, axes rouges, infrastructures lourdes, transport des marchandises par la route ont été systématisés. Le poids des lobbies (routiers, constructeurs automobiles, bétonneurs), qui ont financé les principaux partis politiques, est responsable de cette politique suicidaire.

De plus, les grandes villes sont de plus en plus divisées en zones de travail (le centre), zones d'habitat (les banlieues) et zones de commerce. Paris en est la caricature: les habitants sont expulsés vers la banlieue et 1 million de personnes viennent chaque jour travailler dans la capitale. En 15 ans, les distances parcourues ont doublé, augmentant fortement l'utilisation de l'automobile. **Il faut sortir de l'auto-bureau-dodo.**

Qu'est-il possible de faire?

Il faut commencer par diminuer les risques de crise; doter les villes d'observatoires de surveillance et de prévision de la pollution; informer correctement la population: qu'elle soit prévenue à l'avance des niveaux de pollution, et de leurs conséquences sur la santé. De plus, l'alerte doit être déclenchée dès que des seuils dangereux pour la santé, déterminés par les médecins, sont **prévus**. Enfin, les maires doivent avoir alors l'obligation d'interdire la circulation.

JENNY OLLERENSHAW © 1998, 2002

COLEG LLANDRILLO COLLEGE
LIBRARY RESOURCE CENTRE   077543
CANOLFAN ADNODDAU LLYFRGELL

Au delà, que proposent les Verts?

Nous proposons de limiter la place et les budgets publics accordés à l'automobile et d'augmenter ceux des autres moyens de transport.

Nous proposons de rendre chaque maire juridiquement responsable de la pollution dans sa ville, et de l'adoption d'un Plan de Déplacement Urbain impératif privilégiant les transports en commun, les piétons et les cyclistes, aux dépens de l'automobile. De plus, les agglomérations doivent être progressivement réaménagées pour rapprocher les lieux d'habitat des lieux de travail.

Réorganiser l'espace et les transports prendra des années, **mais si on ne fait rien maintenant, dans 10 ans il sera trop tard.**

Les transports écologiques de demain

Les transports en commun (train, bus, tramway) doivent être massivement aidés, pour devenir conviviaux, bon marché, fiables et rapides, notamment grâce à des voies réservées et protégées.

Les grèves ont montré l'intérêt des citadins pour le vélo et la marche à pied s'ils peuvent circuler en sécurité: dotons les villes de Réseaux Verts (réseaux de rues réservées aux piétons et aux vélos) et de pistes cyclables dignes de ce nom.

Enfin, le transport de marchandises doit être massivement transféré de la route vers le rail.

Laissons la ville respirer, limitons l'automobile!

L'air des villes est de plus en plus pollué à cause de l'automobile. Cette pollution met en danger notre santé: elle est responsable de milliers de morts par an. **Pourtant, la nouvelle loi sur l'air a fait passer les intérêts des lobbies avant la protection de la santé.**

Les Verts proposent de sortir de l' "auto-bureau-dodo"

Limiter la place de l'automobile, favoriser les transports en commun, le transport de marchandises par le rail, le vélo et la marche, rapprocher les lieux de travail des lieux de domicile, doter les villes de Plan de Déplacement Urbain, rendre les maires responsables de la pollution et des interdictions de circulation permettra de diminuer la pollution, d'économiser l'énergie et d'éviter que des millions de personnes perdent chaque jour des heures dans les transports.

Les Verts, Paris

Notes

Les Verts - the main ecologist party in France, founded in 1984. In the June 1997 elections six of their members were elected as députés to the parliament, and one (Madame Dominique Voynet) as a Minister.

6

La Pollution

Exercice 1 ••

Que savez–vous sur la pollution des villes?

Avant de lire le texte lisez les déclarations ci-dessous et essayez de deviner si elles sont vraies ou fausses.

		Vrai	Faux
(a)	Le taux de pollution dans les villes continue à augmenter	☐	☐
(b)	Les industries en France n'ont pas réussi à réduire leur taux de pollution de l'air	☐	☐
(c)	La pollution due à l'automobile n'a pas diminué	☐	☐
(d)	La pollution tue beaucoup de gens chaque année	☐	☐
(e)	Le diesel est un carburant plus propre que l'essence	☐	☐
(f)	La pollution due au diesel peut éventuellement provoquer des cancers	☐	☐
(g)	On essaie depuis 30 ans en France de limiter la place de l'automobile dans la politique des transports	☐	☐
(h)	Les routiers, les constructeurs d'automobiles et les bétonneurs ont beaucoup influencé cette politique des transports	☐	☐
(i)	Le fait que la plupart des gens n'habitent pas près de leur lieu de travail a fortement augmenté l'utilisation de l'automobile	☐	☐

Observations linguistiques

Related words in French and English

The French language is a direct descendant of Latin. Although English is a Germanic language it has many words that come from Norman French, and which therefore could be said to come indirectly from Latin. In English these tend to be 'posh' words that also have more 'down-to-earth' synonyms (often derived from the Germanic or Anglo-Saxon). For example:

Word in English descended from Latin	synonym(s)	French
to annul	to cancel, abolish	annuler
to confound	to confuse, to mix up	confondre
cranium	skull	le crâne
to promulgate	to make known; to promote	promulguer

Although you will not doubt have been warned about **'faux-amis'** (words which look similar in French and English but have a different meaning) there are *far more* **'mots transparents'** (words which look similar and have the same or a very similar meaning) than faux-amis, so do try to guess at the meanings of words that are unfamiliar. The next exercise will give you some practice in this.

JENNY OLLERENSHAW © 1998, 2002

Exercice 2 • • • • • • • • • • • • • • •

Compréhension des mots–clés

1   Lisez d'abord uniquement les sous-titres du texte (par exemple, 'Est-ce dangereux pour la santé?) pour vous donner une idée de son contenu. Ensuite, lisez le texte une fois.

2   Donnez pour chacun des mots 'transparents' de la première colonne au moins un mot en anglais qui lui ressemble et une traduction qui convient dans le contexte. N'utilisez pas votre dictionnaire.

Nous vous avons donné deux exemples:

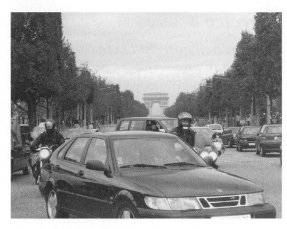

Embouteillages à Paris

mot français du texte	mot qui lui ressemble en anglais	traduction(s) dans le contexte
cesser	to cease	to stop
diminuer	to diminish	to reduce
augmenter		
proliférer		
émettre		
provoquer		
marchandises		
habitat		
expulser		
surveillance		
privilégier		
convivial		
rendre		
permettre		
économiser		

3   Faites de même pour les mots suivants qui demandent un peu plus de réflexion:

mot français du texte	mot qui lui ressemble en anglais	autre(s) traduction(s) possible(s)
incontestablement		
poumons		
cancérigène		
juridiquement		

6

La Pollution

Exercice 3 •

Compréhension du texte

Maintenant que vous avez lu le texte reprenez l'exercice 1 et aidez-vous des informations données dans le texte pour cocher la case 'vrai' ou 'faux'. Si une déclaration est inexacte corrigez-la en français.

Observations linguistiques

The use of the conditional to express a piece of information which is uncertain

Did you notice the use of the conditional in the sentence:

> '... (le diesel) émet des particules fines qui s'accumulent dans les poumons, provoquant des maladies respiratoires et cardio-vasculaires, et qui **seraient** cancérigènes.'

The conditional tense can be used in this way when one cannot fully vouch for the truth of a statement. It is used here because it is thought that the fine particles are carcinogenic, but it has not been proved beyond all doubt.

This use of the conditional is often heard in news bulletins when information about an incident is still coming in and the facts reported have not been fully verified. For example:

> 'Aux dernières nouvelles il y **aurait** deux morts et une dizaine de blessés. Ceux-ci **auraient été** transportés à l'hôpital le plus proche.'

> *Our latest reports **suggest that** there are 2 dead and about 10 injured. These are believed to have been taken to the nearest hospital.*

Note that in English the idea of uncertainty about the facts is not communicated by the tense of the verb, but in this case by the use of the phrases 'to suggest that', and 'are believed to' which also convey the fact that the information may not be totally accurate.

The stylistic omission of 'pas' in a negation

Did you notice the negative:

> '... la pollution due à l'automobile **ne** cesse d'augmenter.'

You may have wondered why there was no 'pas' to go with the first element of the negative 'ne'. In written French 'ne' can be used on its own to express negation with the following verbs: *cesser, oser, pouvoir,* and *savoir.* In such cases the omission of 'pas' makes the phrase sound more elegant.

'Pas' is never used with the verb 'cesser', but in the case of the other verbs 'ne ... pas' could be substituted for the 'ne' without any change in meaning.

Here are some examples of the use of 'ne' on its own:

> Je **n'ose** admettre que ma voiture diesel soit plus polluante qu'une voiture à essence.

> Il est allé s'installer à la campagne. Il **n'aurait pu** faire autrement.

> Je **ne sais** si je dois lui dire que ses enfants risquent de souffrir de crises d'asthme.

> Les voitures **ne cessent** de polluer l'atmosphère.

JENNY OLLERENSHAW © 1998, 2002

Exercice 4 •

Compréhension du texte

Répondez aux questions suivantes en anglais:

1   According to the article what are the first steps that need to be taken?

2   What else do the 'Verts' propose?

3   What plans do they have for public transport?

4   How do they intend to improve the lot of cyclists and pedestrians?

5   What are their plans for the transport of goods?

6   Why are they unhappy with the new legislation on the air?

7   Explain the meaning of the phrase "il faut sortir de l'auto-bureau-dodo".

8   How would their policies help people out of the 'auto-bureau-dodo' trap?

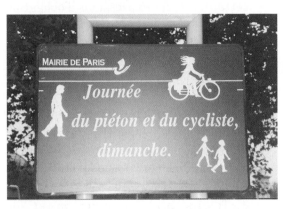

Les citadins feront du vélo et de la marche à pied s'ils peuvent circuler en toute sécurité.

Observations linguistiques

Expressing obligation

Under the paragraph headed 'Qu'est-il possible de faire?' there are two examples of ways to express obligation in French, which will probably be familiar to you:

'Il faut' *(Il faut commencer par diminuer les risques des crise)* and the verb 'devoir' *('l'alerte doit être déclenchée...', 'les maires doivent avoir alors l'obligation d'interdire la circulation')*

There are many other ways of expressing obligation in French. Here are examples of some of them:

Il est obligatoire de respecter la limite de vitesse.
It is compulsory/obligatory to *keep to the speed limit*

Il est indispensable de surveiller le niveau de pollution de l'air
It is essential to *monitor the level of air pollution*

On exige que les habitants des banlieues utilisent les transports en commun
*Commuters **must** use public transport (note that 'exiger que' is followed by the subjunctive)*

Il est stipulé/spécifié que le mode d'emploi doit être écrit en français
It is laid down that *the directions for use be written in French*

Il est nécessaire d'avoir un permis de conduire
It is necessary to *have a driving licence*

Vous êtes obligé de faire une étude plus détaillée sur la question
You have got to *do a more detailed study of the matter*

Il faut absolument ranger les affaires des enfants
You/We really must *tidy the children's things*

Vous devez absolument les mettre en garde contre le danger
You really must *warn them of the danger*

6

La Pollution

Exercice 5 •••••••••••••••

Révision de vocabulaire et de structures

1 Vous allez maintenant réutiliser certaines de ces expressions d'obligation et certains mots et phrases du texte pour traduire les phrases suivantes en français:

a) It will be obligatory to promote public transport to save energy.

b) It is essential to transfer the transport of goods to the railways.

c) It is laid down that the mayors must forbid traffic in town when pollution puts the population in danger.

d) Towns and suburbs **must** be redeveloped to reduce the use of the car.

e) It will be necessary to have a plan which favours public transport.

f) Distances travelled in the car keep on rising. We really must reduce them.

g) There are more and more people who die because of pollution. We have got to make the mayors legally responsible for the pollution in their towns.

h) You must know that air pollution does not only cause respiratory problems.

2 Une fois que vous aurez comparé vos réponses avec celles du corrigé notez et apprenez le vocabulaire et les expressions qui vous ont posé des problèmes pour l'exercice de traduction.

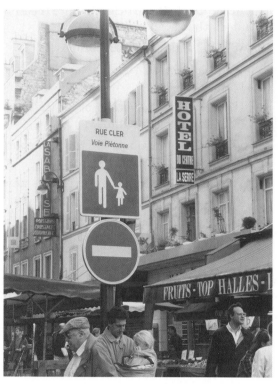

Les voies piétonnes sont essentielles

Exercice 6 ••••••••••••••••••••••••••••••••••

Carnet de notes

Trouvez les mots de liaison ou les expressions suivants dans le texte et notez-les. Vous pourrez ensuite les réutiliser dans vos rédactions ou dans vos discussions en français:

de plus	furthermore/what's more
enfin	finally
grâce à	thanks to
pourtant	all the same, however
dès que	as soon as
aux dépens de	at the expense of
incontestablement	indisputably, unquestionably
à cause de	because of
être dû à	to be due to

Exercice 7 ••••••••••••••

Passage à l'écrit

'Les pays occidentaux doivent absolument limiter la place de l'automobile s'ils ne veulent pas se détruire.'

Relevez dans le texte des exemples qui justifient ce point de vue et donnez en français vos réactions personnelles. N'oubliez pas d'utiliser des mots de liaison.

Ecrivez un maximum de 300 mots.

JENNY OLLERENSHAW © 1998, 2002

6

Corrigés et Explications

Exercice 2 ··

2

mot français du texte	mot qui lui ressemble en anglais	traduction(s) dans le contexte
cesser	to cease	to stop
diminuer	to diminish	to reduce
augmenter	to augment	to increase
proliférer	to proliferate	to increase rapidly/to proliferate
émettre	to emit	to give out
provoquer	to provoke	to cause
marchandises	merchandise	goods
habitat	habitat	living
expulser	to expel	to send/to expel
surveillance	surveillance	monitoring
privilégier	to privilege	to favour/to give priority to
convivial	convivial	friendly
rendre	to render	to make
permettre	to permit	to allow
économiser	to economise	to save

3

mot français du texte	mot qui lui ressemble en anglais	traduction(s) dans le contexte
incontestablement	to contest	indisputably, unquestionably
poumons	pulmonary	lungs
cancérigène	cancer	carcinogenic
juridiquement	jurisdiction, jury	legally

6

Corrigés et Explications

Exercice 3 • • • • • • • • • • • • • • • •

(a) Vrai *'l'air des villes est de plus en plus pollué'*. The air in the cities is more and more polluted.

(b) Faux *'La pollution due aux industries a fortement diminué'*. Industrial pollution has decreased dramatically.

(c) Vrai *'la pollution due à l'automobile ne cesse d'augmenter'*. Pollution from cars keeps on increasing.

(d) Vrai *'L'automobile ... tue aussi des milliers de personnes chaque année par ses pots d'échappement'*. Cars also kill thousands of people each year by their exhausts.

(e) Faux *'le diésel introduit une pollution particulièrement dangereuse'*. Diesel introduces a particularly dangerous form of pollution. (Although pollution from petrol engines is not explicitly compared to that from diesel engines, the implication here is that diesel ones are worse.)

(f) Vrai *'le diésel ... émet des particules fines qui s'accumulent dans les poumons ... et qui seraient cancérigènes'*. Diesel gives out small particles that accumulate in the lungs ... and that are thought to be carcinogenic.

(g) Faux *'Depuis 30 ans la politique des transports se limite au "tout-automobile" ...'*. For 30 years transport policy has been viewed as '**road** transport' policy.

(h) Vrai *'Le poids des lobbies (routiers, constructeurs automobiles, bétonneurs), qui ont financé les principaux partis politiques, est responsable de cette politique suicidaire'*. The influence of the lobbies (truck drivers, car manufacturers and concrete manufacturers), who have financed the main political parties, is responsible for this suicidal policy.

(i) Vrai *'De plus les grandes villes sont divisées en zones de travail ..., zones d'habitat ..., et zones de commerce. Paris en est la caricature: les habitants sont expulsés vers la banlieue et 1 million de personnes viennent chaque jour travailler dans la capitale. En 15 ans, les distances parcourues ont doublé, augmentant fortement l'utilisation de l'automobile'*. What is more the cities are divided into working zones, living zones and shopping zones. Paris is the caricature of this: the inhabitants are expelled to the suburbs and 1 million people come to work every day in the capital. In 15 years, the distances travelled have doubled, greatly increasing the use of the car.

Exercice 4 • • • • • • • • • • • • • • • •

1 The *Verts* suggest that to begin with towns should be equipped with pollution surveillance and forecasting posts. They recommend that the population be kept informed and warned in advance of pollution levels and their health implications. In addition they would like an alert to be given as soon as levels dangerous to health are anticipated (these would be determined by doctors). In such circumstances they would oblige mayors to forbid traffic in the town.

2 They propose restricting the position of the car in order to favour that of other means of transport. Similarly they would also restrict the amount of public money that is spent on cars, in order to increase that spent on other means of transport.

They propose making every mayor legally responsible for the pollution in his/her town, and suggest the adoption of a plan that would favour public transport, pedestrians and cyclists at the expense of cars.

In addition towns and their suburbs would progressively have to be redevelopped in order to bring living areas nearer to working areas.

3 They plan to give massive amounts of aid to public transport (trains, buses, trams) so that they become pleasant, cheap, reliable and fast, in particular thanks to special reserved and protected lanes for them.

4 They say that (transport) strikes have shown that people are interested in using their bicycles or in walking if they can do so in safety. They would like to provide towns with Green Networks (road networks reserved for pedestrians and cyclists) and with cycle lanes which are worthy of their name. (Presumably meaning ones that are reserved **only** for cyclists in practice as well as in theory)

5 They say that the transport of goods must be transferred in a large part from road to rail.

JENNY OLLERENSHAW © 1998, 2002

6 According to them it has put greater emphasis on the interests of lobby groups rather than on the protection of health.

7 'Dodo' is the baby word for 'sleep'. It means that we must escape from the trap of spending one's day travelling in the car to work, doing the day's work, commuting back home in time to go to sleep, only to begin the process again the following day.

8 All of their proposals (listed in the final paragraph) would prevent millions of people from losing hours of their day in travelling.

Exercice 5 • • • • • • • • • • • • • • • • •

a) Il sera obligatoire de favoriser les transports en commun pour économiser l'énergie.

b) Il est indispensable de transférer le transport des marchandises vers le rail/ le chemin de fer.

c) Il est stipulé que les maires doivent interdire la circulation en ville quand la pollution met la population en danger.

d) On exige que les agglomérations soient réaménagées pour réduire l'utilisation de l'automobile. *Did you remember to use the subjunctive after 'on exige que'?*

or Les agglomérations doivent absolument être réaménagées pour réduire l'utilisation de l'automobile.

or Il faut absolument qu'on réaménage les agglomérations pour réduire l'utilisation de l'automobile.

e) Il sera nécessaire d'avoir un plan qui privilégie les transports en commun.

f) Les distances parcourues en voiture ne cessent d'augmenter. Il faut absolument les réduire/Il faut absolument qu'on les réduise. *Did you remember to use 'ne cesse' without the 'pas'?*

g) Il y a de plus en plus de personnes qui meurent à cause de la pollution. On sera obligé de rendre les maires juridiquement responsables de la pollution dans leur ville. *Did you use 'leur ville' rather than the anglicised 'leurs villes'? In French, since each mayor has just one town, the singular is used.*

h) Vous devez savoir que la pollution de l'air ne provoque pas que des maladies respiratoires. *If you had difficulty with translating 'not only' look back at the second paragraph of the text where you had the phrase 'L'automobile ne tue pas que par les accidents'.*

7 L'Association Emmaüs

ACCUEILLIR ET REDONNER ESPOIR

Au coeur d'Emmaüs, il y a une intuition, une conviction: toute personne abandonnée par la société a besoin de se sentir utile aux autres pour redonner un sens à sa vie. Sur cette base sont nées, à partir de 1949, ces communautés d'hommes et de femmes où la dignité de chacun est reconnue. Il pourra y retrouver une identité dans ce milieu de vie qui l'accueille.

L'association Emmaüs est issue de la prise de conscience de personnes militantes qui se sont rassemblées à partir de 1954 autour des idées-forces dont L'Abbé Pierre était porteur, et depuis, l'association Emmaüs n'a jamais cessé de dire et de faire. Dire qu'il est intolérable de laisser une frange de la population en marge de la société, sans toit, ni droit, et depuis quelques années, sans emploi. Que la solidarité ne doit pas seulement être dans tous les discours, mais s'inscrire concrètement dans les choix budgétaires.

Parallèlement, l'association, imprégnée de l'expérience des communautés, met en oeuvre des actions très diversifiées auprès des plus démunis, auprès de ceux que la société rejette. Elle leur offre des lieux d'accueil, toujours animés par cette idée fondamentale: redonner espoir à tous ceux qui en manquent. Redonner espoir, cela signifie aider à faire face aux difficultés de la vie quotidienne. Comment se loger? Comment trouver du travail? Comment percevoir le RMI?

Mais cela ne suffit pas: il faut aussi aider les plus démunis à redonner un sens à leur existence, à trouver des repères et à devenir acteurs de leur vie. Car l'Homme a tout autant besoin d'amour que de nourriture, de dignité que d'un toit, de reconnaissance sociale que de formation et de travail, d'écoute et de considération que de soins médicaux. Depuis son origine, l'association est animée d'un même objectif: offrir un milieu de vie structurant, écouter et accompagner chacun tel qu'il est.

Ce long travail est réalisé par les salariés et les nombreux bénévoles, amis d'Emmaüs. Venant d'horizons les plus divers, ceux-ci jouent un rôle déterminant. Ils sont les jalons, les témoins de rapports humains basés sur la confiance, la réciprocité et l'entraide. Ils permettent la rencontre, le lien social qui est un facteur essentiel de l'insertion.

Cette volonté de faire des ponts est aussi au coeur des pratiques de l'association. Le partenariat n'est pas un vain mot. L'association noue sur des projets précis des collaborations avec des administrations, des collectivités locales – sans que sa liberté de parole en soit entravée. Elle fait pression auprès des gestionnaires du logement (sociétés d'HLM, pouvoirs publics ...) pour qu'ils accueillent les plus démunis. Elle catalyse les énergies de tous ceux qui, dans les entreprises, les associations, les syndicats, le monde culturel, veulent agir pour rendre cette société un peu plus accueillante, fraternelle, et puis, l'association est engagée dans les réflexions et les prises de position d'Emmaüs France.

Ayant toujours refusé de se cantonner dans un rôle gestionnaire, l'association veut interpeller les pouvoirs publics. Pourquoi ne pas ouvrir les centres d'urgence toute l'année, comme nous le demandons depuis des années? Pourquoi la lutte contre l'exclusion est-elle si dépendante de la mobilisation de l'opinion dès les premiers froids?

Dans notre association, chacun (personne accueillie ou celle qui accueille) a sa place. C'est en unissant nos énergies, nos compétences, nos expériences, que nous aiderons ceux qui souffrent à être acteurs de leur réinsertion, mais aussi que nous serons des interlocuteurs efficaces dans le dialogue toujours nécessaire, parfois conflictuel, avec les pouvoirs publics, exerçant ainsi de façon active, notre rôle de citoyen. Car l'association Emmaüs n'est pas seulement le produit d'une immense générosité. C'est aussi le lieu où des citoyens se sont rassemblés

pour exprimer une solidarité réelle, de tous les jours.

Aller plus que jamais à la rencontre de l'autre, l'aider sans l'assister, faire vivre une fraternité de proximité sont les objectifs constants de tous les membres de l'association. Garant de l'idée originelle, le conseil d'administration est le moteur des actions futures. D'où sa volonté de présence au sein des organismes publics ou privés chargés de définir puis de gérer la politique sociale.

Toujours novatrice dans ses moyens d'action, l'association Emmaüs garde son rôle de précurseur sans crainte, si nécessaire, d'être provocatrice.

En cela, l'association Emmaüs reste fidèle à la pensée de son fondateur.

La force du partage, Association Emmaüs, Paris

Notes

L'Association Emmaüs - a charitable organisation which helps the homeless find accommodation and jobs

L'Abbé Pierre - The priest, founder of l'Association Emmaüs, and a well-known and loved figure throughout France

le revenu minimum d'insertion (le RMI) - the minimum benefit paid to those who have no other source of income

trouver des repères - to find points of reference (These could be virtually anything, for example the love of one's family and friends, pride in one's work etc.)

jalons - milestones, markers; here used to describe the rôle of those who work for Emmaüs: they act as firm anchorage points for the homeless

l'aider sans l'assister - help them to help themselves rather than simply doing everything for them, paying for everything etc.

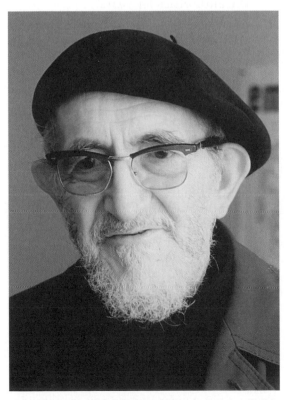

L'Abbé Pierre, fondateur de l'Association Emmaus

Exercice 1 • • • • • • • • • • • • • • •

Compréhension des mots–clés

Lisez le texte en entier sans utiliser de dictionnaire et trouvez l'équivalent français des mots et expressions suivants:

a) resulted from
b) the realisation *(that the problems of the homeless existed)*
c) on the fringes of
d) implements programmes
e) to cope with
f) to receive *(as a benefit)*
g) the most impoverished
h) to take an active role in their own life
i) needs ... as much as ...
j) mutual aid
k) integration
l) without ... being hindered by it
m) to restrict itself
n) administrative
o) hence
p) pioneer

JENNY OLLERENSHAW © 1998, 2002

7

L'Association Emmaüs

Exercice 2 ●●●●●●●●●●●●●●●

Compréhension du texte

Choisissez, pour chacune des phrases suivantes, une fin correcte parmi les trois qui vous sont proposées:

1 C'est l'Abbé Pierre qui
   a) a réalisé par la force les projets des militants
   b) a inspiré les militants par ses idées
   c) a dit qu'il ne faut jamais forcer les militants à accepter ses idées

2 Qu'il y ait des gens qui n'ont pas de logement, pas de travail et pas de droits, l'association Emmaüs trouve cela
   a) inadmissible
   b) incroyable
   c) encourageant

3 L'association Emmaüs
   a) se limite à trouver un logement et un travail pour les plus démunis
   b) pense que la nourriture, le logement, la formation, le travail et les soins médicaux sont les aides les plus importantes à donner aux démunis
   c) considère qu'il est indispensable d'aider les plus démunis à retrouver un sens à leur existence et à prendre des décisions

4 Parmi les gens qui travaillent à l'association
   a) personne ne reçoit de rémunération
   b) il y en a qui sont payés et il y en a qui travaillent sans recevoir de rémunération
   c) la plupart sont payés, très peu travaillent sans recevoir de paiement

5 L'association essaie d'encourager les gestionnaires du logement à
   a) faire pression sur les pouvoirs publics
   b) construire des centres d'accueil pour les démunis
   c) fournir des logements aux démunis

6 A l'association Emmaüs on pense que
   a) les personnes qui sont accueillies ont un rôle très important à jouer dans leur réinsertion
   b) les personnes qui accueillent sont les seules à exercer leur rôle de citoyens
   c) les personnes accueillies ne peuvent pas être des interlocuteurs efficaces face aux pouvoirs publics

7 L'association Emmaüs
   a) veut être représentée dans les organismes qui définissent et gèrent la politique sociale
   b) veut rencontrer plus que jamais les autres organisations caritatives
   c) veut vivre à proximité des organismes publics

8 L'association Emmaüs n'a pas peur de
   a) dépenser l'argent qu'elle gagne
   b) dire ou de faire des choses qui pourraient être mal vues
   c) refuser de l'aide à certains démunis

Exercice 3 ●●●●●●●●●●●●●●●

Compréhension du texte

Répondez en anglais aux questions suivantes:

1 Explain the conviction which is at the heart of the Emmaüs communities and out of which they were born.

2 What does the text say about solidarity and what it means to Emmaüs?

3 How do they define giving back hope to people? How does it go beyond purely practical considerations?

4 Would it be true or not to say that Emmaüs is tied by the fact that it works in partnership with other bodies? Give your reasons.

5 What has Emmaüs been demanding of the authorities for years?

6 In what way is the association true to the spirit of its founder?

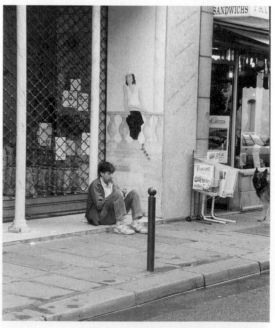

Emmaüs vise à aider ceux qui sont en marge de la société

JENNY OLLERENSHAW © 1998, 2002

Exercice 4 •

Mots croisés

Remplissez ce mots croisés à l'aide des définitions qui suivent. Tous les mots viennent du texte, mais notez que tous les adjectifs dans le mots-croisés sont à la forme masculine.

Ce mots-croisés se lit horizontalement, sauf pour un mot 'caché' vertical (dans les cases en gras) que vous verrez lorsque vous aurez rempli la grille. Ce mot signifie *l'action de rentrer dans la société après en avoir été exclu.*

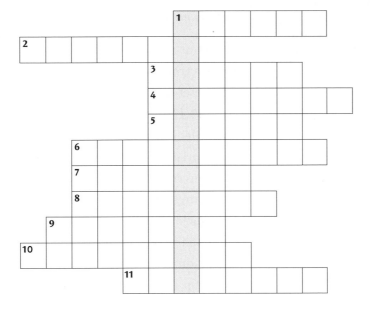

1   un point déterminé qui permet de s'orienter (6)

2   mettre des obstacles, des empêchements à quelque chose (8)

3   loyal (6)

4   aide mutuelle (8)

5   né de (4, 2)

6   confronter (5, 4, 1)

7   personne qui travaille et qui est rémunérée (7)

8   quelqu'un qui innove (8)

9   très pauvres (7)

10 recevoir *(de l'argent)* (9)

11 personne qui travaille sans être rémunérée (8)

7

L'Association Emmaüs

Exercice 5 • • • • • • • • • • • • • • • •

Révision de vocabulaire

Remplissez les blancs dans le texte qui suit avec les mots de l'encadré qui conviennent. Tous les mots sont tirés du texte que vous venez d'étudier.

> l'accueil, démunis, faire face au, centre d'accueil d'urgence, logements, abandonnées, lieu de rencontre, espoir, en marge de, exclusion, mis en oeuvre, prise de conscience, d'accueil, toit, percevoir, d'insertion, faire pression, partenaires, bénévoles, auprès, collaboration, franges, mobiliser

L'Association Emmaüs a été fondée pour _____ problème des personnes _____ par la société, pour _____ auprès des pouvoirs publics pour construire des cités d'urgence et financer des projets en faveur des sans-abri en région parisienne. L'Association est avant tout un _____ pour tous ceux qui, sans distinction de sensibilité politique ou philosophique ou d'appartenance sociale, veulent se _____ contre la misère et la pénurie de _____.

Le travail de milliers de _____ et la _____ de quelques responsables politiques dans les années 50 ont rendu possibles les premiers grands chantiers de construction de logements. Ensuite l'association s'est recentrée sur des activités _____ et d'appui des plus _____ dans leur vie de tous les jours.

Dans les années 70, la crise économique a frappé la France. Des _____ de plus en plus larges de la population ont été touchées. Dans ce contexte, l'association a inventé et a créé de nouvelles structures.

Dans les années 80, la récession économique a frappé de plus en plus les couches populaires. L'association Emmaüs a donc _____ de nouveaux projets. Entre autres, elle a créé un _____ et un vestiaire au Quai de la gare, pour permettre à tous de rester propres et dignes.

Lors du vote de la loi sur le revenu minimum _____, l'association est intervenue _____ des parlementaires pour permettre aux sans-domicile de _____ ce revenu en les domiciliant dans un centre.

Au début des années 90 il y avait en France trois millions de chômeurs et un million et demi de personnes en "grande _____". L'association s'est engagée à travailler en _____ avec des _____ (entreprises, syndicalistes, offices HLM ...) pour ouvrir de nouveaux centres d'urgence. Et le travail de l'association continue. Chaque jour de l'année, l'association Emmaüs se bat avec ses armes à elle - _____ du plus souffrant, le partage - pour redonner un _____ et un _____ à tous les citoyens que les inégalités et les égoïsmes laissent _____ la société.

Exercice 6 • • • • • • • • • • • • • • •

Carnet de notes

Parcourez une dernière fois le texte et notez au moins 12 mots que vous allez apprendre. N'oubliez pas de les noter en contexte.

Exercice 7 • • • • • • • • • • • • • • •

Passage à l'écrit

'Les exclus ont autant besoin de dignité, de reconnaissance sociale et de considération que d'un logement, d'un travail et d'une formation.'

Relevez dans le texte des exemples qui soutiennent ce point de vue et donnez en français vos réactions personnelles.

Ecrivez un maximum de 250 mots.

JENNY OLLERENSHAW © 1998, 2002

Corrigés et Explications

Exercice 1 ● ● ● ● ● ● ● ● ● ● ● ● ● ● ●

a)   resulted from – est issue de

b)   the realisation – la prise de conscience

c)   on the fringes of – en marge de *(Did you get caught out by 'une frange de'? 'Une frange' can mean 'a fringe', but 'une frange de' means 'a minority of'. So here the phrase translates as 'a minority of the population on the fringes of society')*

d)   implements programmes – met en oeuvre des actions

e)   to cope with – faire face à

f)   to receive *(as a benefit)* – percevoir

g)   the most impoverished – les plus démunis

h)   to take an active role in their own life – devenir acteur de leur vie

i)   needs ... as much as ... – a tout autant besoin de ... que de ...

j)   mutual aid– l'entraide

k)   integration– insertion

l)   without ... being hindered by it – sans que ... en soit entravée

m)   to restrict itself – se cantonner

n)   administrative – gestionnaire

o)   hence – d'où

p)   pioneer – précurseur

Exercice 2 ● ● ● ● ● ● ● ● ● ● ● ● ● ●

1   C'était l'Abbé Pierre qui

   b) a inspiré les militants par ses idées

   Para 2: ' ... *la prise de conscience de personnes militantes qui se sont rassemblées ... autour des idées-forces dont l'Abbé Pierre était porteur ...*'

2   Qu'il y ait des gens qui n'ont pas de logement, pas de travail et pas de droits, l'association Emmaüs trouve cela

   a) inadmissible

   Para 2: '... *il est intolérable de laisser une frange de la population en marge de la société ...*'

3   L'association Emmaüs

   c) considère qu'il est indispensable d'aider les plus démunis à retrouver un sens à leur existence et à prendre des décisions

   Para 4: '... *il faut aussi aider les plus démunis à redonner un sens à leur existence, ... et à devenir acteur de leur vie ...*'

4   Parmi les gens qui travaillent à l'association

   b) il y en a qui sont payés et il y en a qui travaillent sans recevoir de rémunération

   Para 5: '*Ce long travail est réalisé par les salariés et les nombreux bénévoles ...*'

5   L'association essaie d'encourager les gestionnaires du logement à

   c) fournir des logements aux démunis

   Para 6: '*Elle fait pression auprès des gestionnaires du logement ... pour qu'ils accueillent les plus démunis*'

6   A l'association Emmaüs on croit que

   a) les personnes qui sont accueillies ont un rôle très important à jouer dans leur réinsertion

   Para 8: '*Dans notre association, chacun (personne accueillie ou celle qui accueille) a sa place. C'est en unissant nos énergies, nos compétences, nos expériences que nous aiderons ceux qui souffrent à être acteurs de leur réinsertion ...*'

7   L'association Emmaüs

   a) veut être représentée dans les organismes qui définissent et gèrent la politique sociale

   Para 9: '*D'où sa volonté de présence au sein des organismes publics ou privés chargés de définir puis de gérer la politique sociale.*'

8   L'association Emmaüs n'a pas peur de

   b) dire ou de faire des choses qui pourraient être mal vues

   Para 10: '... *l'association Emmaüs garde son rôle de précurseur sans crainte, si nécessaire, d'être provocatrice*'

7

Exercice 3 • • • • • • • • • • • • • •

1 The conviction is that everyone who has been abandoned by society needs to feel that they are useful to other people. From this they can begin to find a meaning to their lives again.

Para 1: '... *toute personne abandonnée par la société a besoin de se sentir utile aux autres pour redonner un sens à sa vie.*'

2 Solidarity for them means not just talking about it, but making sure that it is translated into concrete budgetary decisions.

Para 2: '... *la solidarité ne doit pas seulement être dans tous les discours, mais s'inscrire concrètement dans les choix budgétaires.*'

3 For them it means confronting the difficulties of daily life, such as how to find housing, work and how to claim benefits. However, in addition to this, they aim to help the destitute to rediscover the meaning of their lives, to find points of reference and to become active participants in their lives. They believe that people need love as much as food, dignity as much as a roof over their head, social recognition as much as training and work, and someone to listen to and respect them as much as medical care.

Para 3 : '*Redonner espoir, cela signifie ... percevoir le RMI.*'

Para 4: '*Mais cela ne suffit pas ... soins médicaux.*'

4 No. Although they work with other bodies this does not prevent them from expressing their own ideas freely.

Para 6: '... *sans que sa liberté de parole en soit entravée.*'

5 That they open emergency centres all year round: currently the fight against social exclusion is dependent on mobilising public opinion as soon as the bad weather sets in.

Para 7: '*Pourquoi ne pas ouvrir les centres d'urgence toute l'année, comme nous le demandons depuis des années? ...*'

6 It is always innovative in the way that it goes about its work, it maintains its rôle of pioneer, not fearing to be provocative if necessary.

(The whole of Paras 10 & 11)

Exercice 4 •

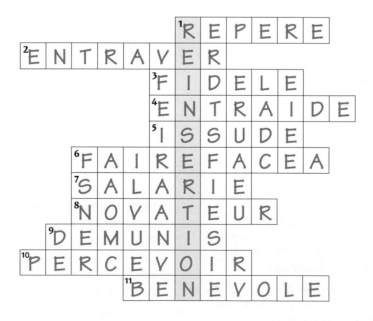

JENNY OLLERENSHAW © 1998, 2002

Exercice 5 • • • • • • • • • • • • • • • •

L'Association Emmaüs a été fondée pour **faire face au** problème des personnes **abandonnées** par la société, pour **faire pression** auprès des pouvoirs publics pour construire des cités d'urgence et financer des projets en faveur des sans-abri en région parisienne. L'Association est avant tout un **lieu de rencontre** pour tous ceux qui, sans distinction de sensibilité politique ou philosophique ou d'appartenance sociale, veulent se **mobiliser** contre la misère et la pénurie de **logement**.

Le travail de milliers de **bénévoles** et la **prise de conscience** de quelques responsables politiques dans les années 50 ont rendu possibles les premiers grands chantiers de construction de logements. Ensuite l'association s'est recentrée sur des activités **d'accueil** et d'appui des plus **démunis** dans leur vie de tous les jours.

Dans les années 70, la crise économique a frappé la France. Des **franges** de plus en plus larges de la population ont été touchées. Dans ce contexte, l'association a inventé et a créé de nouvelles structures.

Dans les années 80, la récession économique a frappé de plus en plus les couches populaires. L'association Emmaüs a donc **mis en oeuvre** de nouveaux projets. Entre autres, elle a créé un **centre d'accueil d'urgence** et un vestiaire au Quai de la gare, pour permettre à tous de rester propres et dignes.

Lors du vote de la loi sur le revenu minimum **d'insertion**, l'association est intervenue **auprès** des parlementaires pour permettre aux sans-domicile de **percevoir** ce revenu en les domiciliant dans un centre.

Au début des années 90 il y avait en France trois millions de chômeurs et un million et demi de personnes en "grande **exclusion**". L'association s'est engagée à travailler en **collaboration** avec des **partenaires** (entreprises, syndicalistes, offices HLM ...) pour ouvrir de nouveaux centres d'urgence. Et le travail de l'association continue. Chaque jour de l'année, l'association Emmaüs se bat avec ses armes à elle - **l'accueil** du plus souffrant, le partage - pour redonner un **toit** et un **espoir** à tous les citoyens que les inégalités et les égoïsmes laissent **en marge de** la société.

Corrigés et Explications

8 Le Chômage et le Racisme

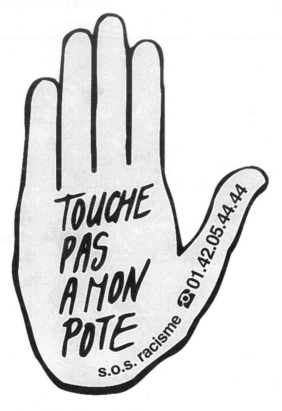

Le célèbre slogan de SOS Racisme

Combattre le Front National

15% aux dernières élections présidentielles, élections municipales de Toulon, Orange et Marignane, implantation dans les syndicats... il ne semble plus y avoir de limites à la progression du Front National. Devenu le premier parti chez les ouvriers, voyant son électorat se populariser et adhérer à son idéologie, la situation du parti lepéniste a changé: nous n'avons plus à faire face à un électorat protestataire et marginal, mais à **un parti structuré qui est candidat au pouvoir.**
Le combat contre le Front National prend donc une nouvelle acuité aujourd'hui. **Chacun de nous se retrouve devant un véritable défi: partir à la reconquête du terrain perdu pour défendre la démocratie...**

JENNY OLLERENSHAW © 1998, 2002

Le Chômage et le Racisme

Chômage

(FN) *"3 millions d'immigrés = 3 millions de chômeurs"*
La logique de ce slogan simpliste implique que les immigrés sont responsables du chômage, c'est-à-dire que s'il n'y avait plus d'immigrés, il n'y aurait plus de chômage.

Ce raisonnement est faux tout d'abord parce que les chiffres sont faux:
– Il n'y a pas "3 millions d'immigrés" en France mais 3,6 millions d'étrangers (la notion d'"immigrés" incluant les Français par naturalisation notamment).
– D'autre part, il n'y a pas "3 millions d'immigrés" qui travaillent. Il faut prendre en compte la seule population active. En effet, un enfant immigré de dix ans ne travaille pas et donc ne prend le travail de personne! De plus, quand le FN parle d'"immigrés", il parle des ressortissants non européens. A l'arrivée, la population concernée par le raisonnement du FN ne représente guère plus de 843 700 étrangers actifs non européens (soit 6,4% de la population active totale en France en incluant les étrangers européens). On est loin des 3 millions de "voleurs d'emplois"...

Il n'y a pas de lien mécanique entre chômage et immigration, les immigrés ne "volent" pas "le travail des Français". En effet, on estime, pour de multiples raisons, que seulement 3 emplois sur 10 occupés par des étrangers pourraient l'être par des Français. Par ailleurs, les immigrés sont plus touchés par le chômage puisqu'il y a 9,5% de Français au chômage contre 18,6% d'étrangers. Ils sont donc également victimes de la crise, et même relativement plus que les Français.

Voilà une des contradictions majeures du programme du FN: il accuse les immigrés à la fois de prendre le travail des Français et en même temps de gonfler les chiffres du chômage. Or on ne peut pas et travailler et être chômeur!

Par ailleurs, le slogan du Front National, qui vise à faire des immigrés les boucs-émissaires de la crise, n'est pas sans rappeler le "3 millions de juifs = 3 millions de chômeurs" scandé par les nazis en Allemagne dans les années 30.

(FN) *"Les immigrés profitent du chômage"*
Le chômage serait en partie le résultat de l'ouverture de nos frontières à l'immigration et de mécanismes sociaux protecteurs garantissant un minimum de revenus aux salariés privés d'emplois. C'est-à-dire que notre système d'allocation-chômage profiterait aux étrangers qui viendraient ainsi gonfler artificiellement la masse des chômeurs.

Il convient de rappeler que **ne perçoivent des prestations chômage, que les immigrés ayant précédemment cotisé et donc travaillé en France.**
Ces prestations ne sont qu'une forme légitime de salaire différé correspondant à ce qu'ils n'ont pas touché lorsqu'ils cotisaient, et ce comme pour tous les autres travailleurs. D'autre part, les immigrés ne "profitent" pas tant que ça de notre système puisque les travailleurs immigrés non-européens touchent des prestations inférieures à celles des Français. Ainsi, on estime qu'environ 35% des étrangers hors CEE ne touchent aucune indemnité contre 28% en moyenne, tandis que 34% d'entre eux touchent une allocation inférieure à 2 000F par mois.

Ⓕⓝ *"Priorité d'emploi aux Français"*
Pour garantir la priorité d'emploi aux Français, le FN propose plusieurs mesures, notamment au niveau des conditions d'embauche (priorité aux Français) et de licenciement (priorité aux immigrés), la plus extrême de ces mesures consistant "tout simplement" à renvoyer les immigrés d'où ils viennent, pour être plus sûr qu'ils ne prennent pas l'emploi des Français et qu'ils ne leur coûtent pas un centime...

Outre le fait que ces expulsions dégageraient relativement peu d'emplois car **il n'y a pas de lien mécanique entre immigration et chômage**, cette mesure aurait des effets pervers désastreux: l'expulsion des immigrés et de leurs familles entraînerait une contraction importante de la demande sur le marché intérieur, ce qui génèrerait un surcroît de chômage (des millions de consommateurs en moins, ...).

Certes les immigrés ont des devoirs, mais ils ont aussi des droits, ce sont des travailleurs comme les autres, ils paient des impôts, des cotisations sociales, participent au développement de l'entreprise et ce au même titre que les autres travailleurs... **ils doivent donc être traités avec les mêmes égards**. D'autant plus que de nombreux immigrés ont participé à l'essor économique de notre pays, notamment durant la période des Trente Glorieuses.

Ⓕⓝ *"Il faut taxer le travail immigré"*
Pour pénaliser les entrepreneurs au comportement "anti-français" qui emploient des immigrés, le FN propose d'instituer une taxe les pénalisant systématiquement.

Cette proposition constitue une véritable atteinte à la liberté des individus mais elle est surtout dénuée de tout fondement dans la mesure où **un travailleur contribue au rayonnement de notre pays non pas en fonction de sa nationalité mais en fonction de la qualité de son travail.** On ne peut donc pas dire qu'employer un immigré relève d'un comportement "anti-français".

De plus, cette mesure n'est pas sans rappeler la teneur des lois antijuives, mises en place par le gouvernement de Vichy pendant l'occupation allemande, qui interdisaient aux juifs l'exercice de certaines professions.

'Défendre la Démocratie! 50 réponses au programme du Front National', 1996, SOS Racisme, Paris

Notes

le parti lepéniste - The far-right political party, le 'Front National' (FN), led by Jean-Marie Le Pen

les Trente Glorieuses - the three decades between the end of the Second World War and the mid-1970s during which France saw sustained economic growth and social transformation (the expression is a pun on *les Trois Glorieuses* - the three days of revolution from 27th to 29th July 1830 which led to the abdication of King Charles X)

Le texte que vous allez lire est tiré d'un document publié par l'association 'SOS Racisme' qui s'appelle *"Défendre la Démocratie! 50 réponses au programme du Front National"*. Fondée en 1984, cette association a pour but de lutter contre le racisme en France. Ce texte de 'SOS Racisme' contient quelques citations (précédées du sigle FN entouré d'un cercle) qui sont issues du programme du 'Front National' *"300 mesures pour la renaissance de la France"* (1993) ainsi que de son matériel de propagande électorale lors des élections présidentielles en 1995. Le commentaire qui suit et qui se trouve à côté de la main 'touche pas à mon pote!' (le badge de l'association) est celui de l'association 'SOS Racisme'.

JENNY OLLERENSHAW © 1998, 2002

Exercice 1 •••

Compréhension des mots–clés

Lisez une fois le texte en entier sans vous aider du dictionnaire. Le but de cette première lecture sera de comprendre quelques mots-clés liés au chômage. Dans le tableau-ci dessous, ils sont dans la colonne de gauche dans l'ordre où ils apparaissent dans le texte (ils sont tous tirés de la deuxième moitié du texte). Les définitions de ces mots sont en vrac dans la colonne de droite. Trouvez la définition qui correspond à chaque mot. Attention, il y a deux mots qui, dans le contexte du chômage, ont la même définition.

mot du texte	définition
percevoir	verser régulièrement une somme d'argent
des prestations chômage	somme versée par le gouvernement à un individu pour faire face à un besoin
cotiser	rupture (à l'initiative de l'employeur) d'un contrat de travail
une indemnité	recevoir (de l'argent)
une allocation	offre de travail
l'embauche	part du salaire que chaque personne qui travaille doit payer à l'Etat
le licenciement	somme versée par le gouvernement à un individu pour faire face à un besoin
les impôts	argent versé à l'Etat par un travailleur et qui sert à couvrir les frais de sécurité sociale
les cotisations sociales	sommes d'argent versées aux chômeurs par le gouvernement

Exercice 2 •••

Compréhension des mots–clés

Maintenant regardez la liste de bouts de phrases tirés du texte. Pour chacun d'eux choisissez parmi les trois paraphrases données celle qui lui correspond le mieux:

1   *le combat ... prend donc une nouvelle acuité*

   a) le combat devient plus intense

   b) on cherche de nouveaux adhérents pour le combat

   c) le combat devient de plus en plus difficile

2   *partir à la reconquête du terrain perdu*

   a) essayer de racheter du terrain pour construire des maisons pour les immigés

   b) essayer de renverser les victoires du 'Front National' aux dernières élections

   c) essayer d'expliquer aux lepénistes que la démocratie n'est pas perdue

3   *les Français par naturalisation*

   a) les étrangers auxquels on a accordé la nationalité française

   b) les Français qui ont la double nationalité

   c) les Français qui sont nés à l'étranger

4   *les ressortissants non-européens*

   a) les Français qui sont nés hors de la Communauté Européenne

   b) les travailleurs non-européens

   c) les citoyens de pays non-européens

JENNY OLLERENSHAW © 1998, 2002

8

Le Chômage et le Racisme

5 *(le FN) accuse les immigrés ... de gonfler les chiffres du chômage*

   a) s'il n'y avait pas autant d'immigrés au chômage le nombre de chômeurs en France serait beaucoup plus bas

   b) les immigrés touchent les allocations de chômage sans en avoir le droit

   c) le coût des allocations de chômage est très élevé à cause des chômeurs immigrés

6 *... qui vise à faire des immigrés les boucs-émissaires de la crise*

   a) qui essaye de taxer les immigrés pour aider la France à sortir de la crise

   b) qui tente de faire que les plus touchés par la crise soient les immigrés

   c) qui essaye de faire des immigrés les responsables de la crise

7 *(les) salariés privés d'emplois*

   a) les salariés qui travaillent dans le secteur privé

   b) les salariés qui ont perdu leur emploi

   c) les salariés qui cherchent un emploi privé

8 *l'expulsion des immigrés ... générerait un surcroît de chômage*

   a) suite aux expulsions, il y aurait encore plus de chômeurs

   b) suite aux expulsions, il y aurait sûrement moins de chômeurs

   c) les expulsions n'auraient en général aucun effet sur le taux de chômage

9 *les immigrés ... participent au développement de l'entreprise ... au même titre que les autres travailleurs*

   a) les immigrés qui participent au développement de l'entreprise ont le même droit au travail que les autres travailleurs

   b) les immigrés participent davantage au développement de l'entreprise que les autres travailleurs

   c) les immigrés participent au développement de la production tout comme les autres travailleurs

10) *de nombreux immigrés ont participé à l'essor économique de notre pays*

   a) Beaucoup d'immigrés ont contribué à la crise économique que subit la France

   b) Les immigrés sont responsables de la crise économique en France

   c) beaucoup d'immigrés ont joué un rôle dans l'expansion économique de la France

Exercice 3 • • • • • • • • • • • • • • • • •

Compréhension du texte

Répondez aux questions suivantes en français. Dans la mesure du possible, essayez d'utiliser vos propres mots au lieu de reprendre les mots du texte.

1 Dans quelle mesure l'idée que l'on se fait du parti lepéniste a-t-elle changé depuis les dernières élections présidentielles et municipales?

2 Expliquez ce qu'implique le slogan du 'Front National': "3 millions d'immigrés = 3 millions de chômeurs".

3 Selon 'SOS Racisme', pourquoi cet argument est-il faux?

4 Selon 'SOS Racisme', quel pourcentage d'emplois occupés actuellement par des étrangers pourraient être occupés par des Français?

5 Selon 'SOS Racisme' quelle est l'une des contradictions majeures du programme du 'Front National'?

6 A quoi 'SOS Racisme' compare-t-il la réaction du 'Front National' au chômage?

7 Selon le 'Front National', quelle est la politique qui encourage les immigrés à profiter du chômage?

8 Quel est l'argument de 'SOS Racisme' contre la prétention que le système d'allocation chômage profite aux étrangers?

9 Selon 'SOS Racisme', pourquoi l'expulsion des immigrés serait-elle contre-productive pour la France?

10 D'après 'SOS Racisme' pourquoi n'y a-t-il aucun sens à taxer le travail immigré?

JENNY OLLERENSHAW © 1998, 2002

Observations linguistiques

The use of the conditional to refer to a possible future

You have no doubt come across the use of the conditional following a 'si' clause to express a possible future outcome. Look at this example from the text:

'... c'est à dire que s'il n'y **avait** plus d'immigrés, il n'y **aurait** plus de chômage.'

*That is to say that if there **were** no more immigrants there **would be** no more unemployment.*

Note that in this type of sentence the verb in the 'si' clause is in the *imperfect* and the verb in the clause expressing the possible outcome is in the *conditional*. The following exercise will give you the chance to revise this type of sentence.

Exercice 4 •••

Révision du conditionnel

En choisissant le début d'une phrase de la colonne de gauche et la fin d'une phrase de la colonne de droite reconstituez autant de phrases que possible qui auraient pu être prononcées par le 'Front National' ou par 'SOS Racisme' au sujet des immigrés et du chômage. Ensuite signalez laquelle des deux organisations aurait pu prononcer la phrase. Pour chaque phrase vous devez conjuguer les verbes donnés à l'infinitif.

Exemple:

la France ne pas (garantir) l'allocation chômage	on (avoir) moins de chômeurs étrangers en France.

Si la France ne garantissait pas l'allocation chômage on aurait moins de chômeurs étrangers en France. (FN)

on (expulser) tous les immigrés	il (voir) que les étrangers sont plus touchés par la crise que les Français
le 'Front National' (tenir) compte des immigrés qui ne travaillent pas	il y (avoir) davantage de chômage
le 'Front National'(regarder) de près les statistiques	ils (avoir) droit à une indemnité plus élevée
les immigrés ne pas (avoir) cotisé et travaillé en France	il y (avoir) plus d'emplois pour les Français
les chômeurs (avoir) la nationalité française	on (nuire) au rayonnement de la France
on (pénaliser) les entrepreneurs qui emploient des immigrés	on (pénaliser) les entrepreneurs qui emploient les immigrés
on (arriver) au pouvoir	ils ne pas (avoir) droit à l'allocation chômage
	il (constater) qu'il n'y a que 843 700 étrangers actifs non européens en France
	il y (avoir) une contraction importante sur le marché intérieur ce qui (générer) un surcroît de chômage

8

Observations linguistiques

The use of the conditional to imply conjecture or allegation

In French the conditional tense can be used when one cannot fully vouch for the truth of a statement. So, for instance, it is often used in news bulletins when information about an incident is still coming in and the facts reported have not been fully verified. For example:

'Il y a eu un accident de route: il y **aurait** cinq blessés'

*There has been a road accident: there are **thought to be** five wounded*

Note that in English the idea of uncertainty about the facts is not communicated by the tense of the verb, but in this case by the use of the phrase 'there are thought to be', which also conveys the fact that the information may not be totally accurate.

In the text, under the heading **"les immigrés profitent du chômage"** 'SOS Racisme' explains what the 'Front National' means by this, but distances themselves from the explanation by the use of the conditional, which shows that they do not think that what the 'Front National' says on the matter is true:

'Le chômage **serait** en partie le résultat de l'ouverture de nos frontières à l'immigration ... notre système d'allocation-chômage **profiterait** aux étrangers qui **viendraient** ainsi gonfler artificiellement la masse des chômeurs.'

*Unemployment **is alleged to be** partly the result of the opening of our borders to immigration ... our system of unemployment benefit **is seen** (by the 'Front National') to benefit foreignors who, **they claim,** come here and artificially swell the ranks of the unemployed.*

Prepositions

In French some verbs or phrases are always followed by a particular prepostion (for example, 'de', 'à', 'par', 'entre'). It is very important to learn the preposition at the same time as you learn the verb or phrase. This text has many such examples, and the next two activities will help you identify them and learn them by using them.

Exercice 5 ··

Repérage des prépositions

Voici la liste de tous les verbes et expressions suivis des prépositions 'de', 'à', 'par' ou 'entre'. Avant de regarder le texte de nouveau essayez de noter la préposition qui, d'après vous, suit le verbe ou l'expression. Ensuite vérifiez votre travail en vous référant au texte.

adhérer

faire face

être candidat

être responsable

être concerné

être loin

il y a un lien

être occupé

être touché

viser

être le résultat

être privé

il convient

correspondre

profiter

consister

coûter de l'argent __ (quelqu'un)

participer

proposer

être dénué

en fonction

relever

interdire __ (quelqu'un)

JENNY OLLERENSHAW © 1998, 2002

Exercice 6 • • • • • • • • • • • • • •

Choix de la bonne préposition

Complétez les phrases suivantes en insérant la préposition qui convient. N'oubliez pas de faire les changements nécessaires (par exemple: de → des, à → aux etc.) et essayez de faire l'exercice sans regarder vos notes.

1   Il propose ____ participer ____ les frais du voyage.

2   Ce politique est totalement dénué ____ scrupules. Ses décisions vont coûter une fortune ____ les consommateurs.

3   J'adhère ____ l'opinion que la France ne devrait pas établir une discrimination envers les immigrés.

4   Notre région était très touchée ____ la sécheresse.

5   Il profite honteusement ____ ta générosité! Tu dois faire face ____ la réalité avant qu'il ne soit trop tard.

6   Elle sera candidate ____ les prochaines élections municipales.

7   Ce que vous me racontez ne correspond pas du tout ____ ce que j'avais imaginé.

8   La maison d'à côté est occupée ____ une famille marocaine.

9   Le campagne publicitaire vise ____ changer l'attitude des gens.

10 Je me sens très concernée ____ cette décision.

11 Je suis responsable ____ cette situation et j'interdis ____ tout le monde d'en parler à qui que ce soit.

12 Leur programme consiste ____ aider ceux qui sont privés ____ logement et ____ travail.

13 Il convient ____ rappeler que l'on est loin de trouver une solution ____ cette crise.

14 'Il n'y a aucun lien ____ votre licenciement et le fait que vous avez fait grève. C'est le résultat ____ longues discussions.'

15 Ce n'est pas à moi qu'il faut s'adresser. Cela relève ____ le Ministère de l'Environnement.

16 Vous recevrez un salaire en fonction ____ votre expérience.

Exercice 7 •

Carnet de notes

Trouvez dans le texte les mots de liaison suivants et notez-les. Vous pourrez ensuite les réutiliser dans vos rédactions ou dans vos discussions en français:

d'autre part	moreover
en effet	indeed, actually
de plus	moreover
à l'arrivée	at the end of the day
on estime que	it is considered that
par ailleurs	in addition
puisque	since
donc	therefore
or	and yet
il convient de rappeler que	it should be remembered that
ainsi	thus
outre	as well as, in addition to
certes	admittedly
d'autant plus que	all the more so since

8

Le Chômage et le Racisme

Exercice 8 • • • • • • • • • • • • • •

Passage à l'écrit

'Le "Front National" a tort de dire que les immigrés sont responsables du chômage en France.'

Relevez dans le texte des arguments qui justifient ce point de vue et donnez en français vos réactions personnelles. N'oubliez pas d'utiliser des mots de liaison là où il convient.

Ecrivez un maximum de 320 mots.

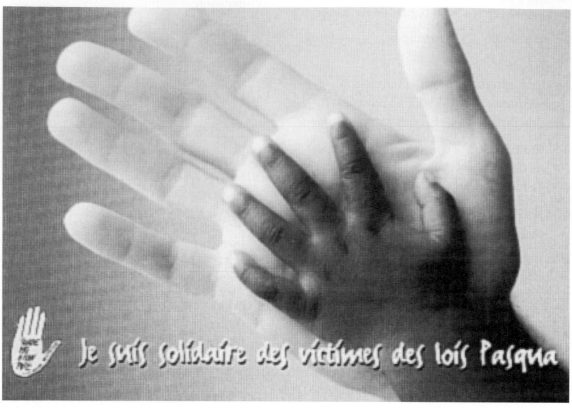

'SOS Racisme' lutte contre toutes manifestations du racisme

JENNY OLLERENSHAW © 1998, 2002

Corrigés et Explications

Exercice 1

mot du texte	définition
percevoir	recevoir (de l'argent)
des prestations chômage	sommes d'argent versées aux chômeurs par le gouvernement
cotiser	verser régulièrement une somme d'argent
une indemnité	somme versée par le gouvernement à un individu pour faire face à un besoin
une allocation	somme versée par le gouvernement à un individu pour faire face à un besoin
l'embauche	offre de travail
le licenciement	rupture (à l'initiative de l'employeur) d'un contrat de travail
les impôts travaille doit payer à l'Etat	part du salaire que chaque personne qui
les cotisations sociales	argent versé à l'Etat par un travailleur et qui sert à couvrir les frais de sécurité sociale

Exercice 2

1 le combat ... prend donc une nouvelle acuité

a) le combat devient plus intense

2 partir à la reconquête du terrain perdu

b) essayer de renverser les victoires du 'Front National' aux dernières élections

3 les Français par naturalisation

a) les étrangers auxquels on a accordé la nationalité française

4 les ressortissants non européens

c) les citoyens de pays non européens

5 (le FN) accuse les immigrés ... de gonfler les chiffres du chômage

a) s'il n'y avait pas autant d'immigrés au chômage le nombre de chômeurs en France serait beaucoup plus bas

6 ... qui vise à faire des immigrés les boucs-émissaires de la crise

c) qui essaye de faire des immigrés les responsables de la crise

7 (les) salariés privés d'emplois

b) les salariés qui ont perdu leur emploi

8 l'expulsion des immigrés ...générerait un surcroît de chômage

a) suite aux expulsions il y aurait encore plus de chômeurs

9 les immigrés ... participent au développement de l'entreprise ... au même titre que les autres travailleurs

c) les immigrés participent au développement de la production tout comme les autres travailleurs

10 de nombreux immigrés ont participé à l'essor économique de notre pays

c) beaucoup d'immigrés ont joué un rôle dans l'expansion économique de la France

8

Corrigés et Explications

Exercice 3 ••••••••••••••••

Here are our suggested answers. Yours will no doubt differ in expression, but make sure that the sense is the same.

1 Avant ces élections les gens qui votaient pour le 'Front National' étaient considérés comme des marginaux qui protestaient, mais maintenant que le parti a obtenu autant de votes on considère que c'est un parti structuré qui pourrait éventuellement arriver au pouvoir un jour.

2 Le 'Front National' prétend que s'il n'y avait pas 3 millions d'immigrés en France il y aurait 3 millions d'emplois en plus pour les Français qui sont actuellement au chômage.

3 Parce que le 'Front National' ne tient pas compte de tous les immigrés qui ne travaillent pas (par exemple les enfants et les chômeurs). 'SOS Racisme' explique qu'il n'y a que 843 700 'immigrés' qui travaillent en France, et non pas 3 millions.

4 33.3% (3 sur 10)

5 Le 'Front National' accuse les immigrés de prendre le travail des Français. Il les accuse aussi de constituer une grande proportion des chômeurs en France. 'SOS Racisme' fait remarquer que les mêmes personnes ne peuvent être travailleurs et chômeurs en même temps.

6 Il la compare au slogan qu'on entendait dans les années 30 en Allemagne, où les Nazis scandaient: "3 millions de juifs=3 millions de chômeurs".

7 Celle qui est pour l'ouverture des frontières de la France à l'immigration et pour la garantie d'un minimum de revenus aux salariés qui sont privés d'emploi.

8 Ce sont seulement les immigrés qui ont payé leurs cotisations en France (ce qui prouve qu'ils ont travaillé) qui peuvent bénéficier des allocations chômage. Donc ils n'en 'profitent' pas: ils y ont droit. En plus ils font remarquer qu'en France le montant de l'allocation-chômage est moins élevé pour un chômeur non européen que pour un chômeur français.

9 a) Selon 'SOS Racisme' l'expulsion ne dégagerait pas beaucoup d'emplois (seulement 33.3% des emplois tenus par des immigrés pourraient être occupés par des Français - voir la question 4)

b) Si les immigrés et leurs familles étaient expulsés il y aurait beaucoup moins de consommateurs en France, ce qui créerait encore plus de chômage.

10 'SOS Racisme' soutient que ce qui détermine la contribution d'un travailleur à la réussite d'un pays c'est la qualité de son travail et non pas sa nationalité.

Exercice 4 ••••••••••••••••

Here are our suggestions. Check the form of your verbs carefully with ours to make sure that you have used the correct form of the verb.

Si on expulsait tous les immigrés il y aurait une contraction importante sur le marché intérieur, ce qui générerait un surcroît de chômage. *'SOS Racisme'*

Si on expulsait tous les immigrés il y aurait davantage de chômage. *'SOS Racisme'*

Si on expulsait tous les immigrés il y aurait plus d'emplois pour les Français. *Le 'Front National'*

Si le 'Front National' tenait compte des immigrés qui ne travaillent pas il constaterait qu'il n'y a que 843 700 étrangers actifs non européens en France. *'SOS Racisme'*

Si le 'Front National' regardait de près les statistiques il verrait que les étrangers sont plus touchés par la crise que les Français. *'SOS Racisme'*

Si le 'Front National' regardait de près les statistiques il constaterait qu'il n'y a que 843 700 étrangers actifs non-européens en France. *'SOS Racisme'*

Si un immigré n'avait pas cotisé et travaillé en France il n'aurait pas droit à l'allocation chômage. *'SOS Racisme'*

Si les chômeurs avaient la nationalité française ils auraient droit à une indemnité plus élevée. *'SOS Racisme'*

Si on pénalisait les entrepreneurs qui emploient des immigrés on nuirait au rayonnement de la France. *'SOS Racisme'*

Si on pénalisait les entrepreneurs qui emploient des immigrés il y aurait plus d'emplois pour les Français. *Le 'Front National'*

Si on arrivait au pouvoir on pénaliserait les entrepreneurs qui emploient des immigrés. *Le 'Front National'*

Si on arrivait au pouvoir il y aurait plus d'emplois pour les Français. *Le 'Front National'*

JENNY OLLERENSHAW © 1998, 2002

Exercice 5 •

verbe/expression + 'à'	verbe/expression + 'de'
adhérer à	être responsable de
faire face à	être loin de
être candidat à	être le résultat de
viser à	être privé de
correspondre à	il convient de
consister à	profiter de
coûter de l'argent à (quelqu'un)	proposer de
participer à	être dénué de
interdire à (quelqu'un)	en fonction de
	relever de

verbe/expression + 'par'	verbe/expression + 'entre'
être concerné par	il y a un lien entre
être occupé par	
être touché par	

Exercice 6 • • • • • • • • • • • • • • •

1   Il propose de participer **aux** frais du voyage.

2   Ce politique est totalement dénué **de** scrupules. Ses décisions vont coûter une fortune **aux** consommateurs.

3   J'adhère **à** l'opinion que la France ne devrait pas établir une discrimination envers les immigrés.

4   Notre région était très touchée **par** la sécheresse.

5   Il profite honteusement **de** ta générosité! Tu dois faire face **à** la réalité avant qu'il ne soit trop tard.

6   Elle sera candidate **aux** prochaines élections municipales.

7   Ce que vous me racontez ne correspond pas du tout **à** ce que j'avais imaginé.

8   La maison d'à côté est occupée **par** une famille marocaine.

9   Le campagne publicitaire vise **à** changer l'attitude des gens.

10   Je me sens très concernée **par** cette décision.

11   Je suis responsable **de** cette situation et j'interdis **à** tout le monde d'en parler à qui que ce soit.

12   Leur programme consiste **à** aider ceux qui sont privés **de** logement et **de** travail.

13   Il convient **de** rappeler que l'on est loin de trouver une solution **à** cette crise.

14   'Il n'y a aucun lien **entre** votre licenciement et le fait que vous avez fait grève. C'est le résultat **de** longues discussions.'

15   Ce n'est pas à moi qu'il faut s'adresser. Cela relève **du** Ministère de l'Environnement.

16   Vous recevrez un salaire en fonction **de** votre expérience.

Model Essays

Model Essays

Unit 1 – Le Recyclage

'Pour inverser le processus actuel de pollution de notre environement il n'est pas question d'employer de demi-mesures.' Relevez dans le texte des exemples qui justifient ce point de vue et donnez en français vos réactions personnelles.

Écrivez environ 150 mots.

La France, qui compte aujourd'hui presque 60 millions d'habitants, 'produirait' 80 millions de tonnes de déchets par an! Parmi ceux-ci 18 millions de tonnes sont qualifiés de 'déchets ménagers' dont 45 % sont uniquement constitués par les emballages qui ne sont ni recyclables ni biodégradables.

Certes, des efforts ont été accomplis dans le tri sélectif mais il est plus que nécessaire aujourd'hui de s'engager sans tergiversations dans une lutte totale en refusant les demi-mesures: car l'effet de serre généré par les émanations de gaz et la pollution de l'air et de l'eau causée par les déchets fermentescibles ne font que s'aggraver, mettant en péril peu à peu tout l'équilibre de notre planète.

Il faut donc absolument inverser le processus actuel de pollution. Je suis convaincu(e) que l'enjeu est à la mesure des défis que l'homme peut et doit relever à l'aube du XXIe siècle.

Unit 2. Les Sans Domicile Fixe

'L'État français n'accepte pas ses responsabilités envers les plus démunis de la société.' Relevez dans le texte des exemples qui justifient ce point de vue et donnez en français vos réactions personnelles.

Écrivez un maximum de 200 mots.

En France, les personnes appartenant aux catégories de population défavorisées, telles que les jeunes sans emploi et sans allocations, les chômeurs en fin de droits, (dont les allocations diminuent mois après mois) les étrangers arrivés sans papiers, (et donc sans autorisation de séjour) et les SDF, ont 'officiellement' le droit d'être soignées gratuitement dans les hôpitaux et les dispensaires. Ce droit est bien inscrit dans la loi française.

Cependant, dans une société très formelle et réglementée, ces personnes qualifiées de 'marginales' restent hélas à l'écart du système général de santé. En effet, excepté dans les services d'Urgences, où tout individu gravement malade ou accidenté entre sans formalité, les hôpitaux et dispensaires sont trop structurés pour l'étranger qui ne parle pas bien français. Celui-ci ne saura pas expliquer sa maladie, ni remplir un document. Il en sera de même pour le SDF qui ne pourra fournir aucune adresse et pour le 'sans papiers' dont la précarité est plus grande encore…

Heureusement, les Centres de soins et d'hébergement médicalisé, mis en place depuis 1989 par Médecins Sans Frontières à l'intention de tous ces exclus, ont ouvert une nouvelle voie pour assurer à tous le droit à la santé. On ne peut qu'applaudir cette mesure.

JENNY OLLERENSHAW © 1998, 2002

COLEG LLANDRILLO COLLEGE
LIBRARY RESOURCE CENTRE
CANOLFAN ADNODDAU LLYFRGELL

Unit 3. L'Alcoolisme

'L'alcoolisme est une vraie maladie, souvent jugée 'infamante', mais que l'on peut arriver à soigner.' Relevez dans le texte des exemples qui justifient ce point de vue et donnez, en français, vos rézctions personnelles.

Écrivez un maximum de 250 mots.

La recherche médicale progresse dans les domaines les plus divers. Cependant, en dépit des moyens mis en œuvre, et des découvertes scientifiques, certaines pathologies comportementales restent difficiles à soigner: ainsi, l'alcoolisme, toujours considéré comme une honte, qui marque le malade lui-même, mais également sa famille.

C'est la raison pour laquelle, la personne devenue dépendante de l'alcool refuse souvent de reconnaître son problème, né d'un contexte circonstanciel plus ou moins long et d'événements vécus, dont la gravité est toujours subjective. Il est évident que, pour aider cette personne à se débarrasser de cette 'drogue', un ancien alcoolique sera le meilleur soutien, car il a lui aussi connu la dépendance de plus en plus profonde à l'alcool, sa domination, la difficulté d'évoquer son problème avec ses proches ou seulement d'accepter le diagnostic d'un médecin. L'important, il me semble, est d'intervenir aussitôt que possible, c'est à dire avant que le malade perde le contrôle sur sa consommation et surtout avant qu'il connaisse troubles graves et délabrement physique. En fait, il faut absolument empêcher que le malade se renferme sur lui-même. En effet, devenu incapable de combattre seul son penchant, il sera dans l'impossibilité d'arrêter un processus, qui deviendra irréversible.

Encouragé par son entourage proche et par des personnes qui ont surmonté la même dépendance, un alcoolique a toutes les chances de s'en sortir s'il admet la nécessité de rompre complètement avec une attirance qui, en fait, n'a que des effets négatifs.

Unit 4. Le Nucléaire et la Santé.

Reprenez les notes que vous avez prises pour l'exercice 2, ainsi que le corrigé de cet exercice. A l'aide de ces notes écrivez un court article sur les recherches sur les risques de leucémie, les groupes à risque et les mesures qui vont être prises suite au débat. Essayez de réutiliser le vocabulaire que vous avez appris ainsi que les mots de liaison qui conviennent.

Écrivez un maximum de 200 mots.

Les plus récentes études menées, tant en France qu'en Grande-Bretagne, à propos des risques épidémiologiques encourus par les populations proches des installations nucléaires, ont révélé un taux important de leucémies touchant particulièrement les enfants.

En France, des prélèvements ont été effectués à proximité de La Hague, dans la presqu'île du Cotentin où le vaste complexe industriel de la COGEMA procède au retraitement de combustibles nucléaires usés (après séparation d'avec les produits de fission fortement radioactifs). Des 'éléments convaincants' sont venus confirmer une première étude, menée en 1995, cette fois-là en Grande-Bretagne, parmi les populations proches des sites nucléaires de Sellafield et Dounreay. La fréquentation des plages, mais aussi la consommation (à raison seulement d'une fois par semaine) de poissons et crustacés pêchés dans ces zones, ont démontré des risques majeurs de contamination.

Ces résultats concordants ne font toutefois pas l'unanimité et des études complémentaires indépendantes devraient permettre d'étayer ou d'infirmer les thèses en présence. Les risques, s'ils existent, seraient ainsi clairement établis. Les responsables politiques ou économiques pourraient alors engager, en toute connaissance de causes, les actions qui s'imposent pour assurer la sécurité des populations.

Model Essays

Model Essays

Unit 5. L'Euthanasie

Écrivez une rédaction de 200 à 250 mots dans laquelle vous expliquerez pourquoi vous êtes pour ou contre l'euthanasie. Essayez de réutiliser les expressions et le vocabulaire que vous avez vus dans le texte.

Nous savons tous que notre mort est inscrite dans notre condition d'humains et je suis convaincu(e) qu'il faut accepter l'idée de la mort comme on accepte celle de la vie puisque nous n'avons pas eu non plus le 'choix de naître'. Prendre conscience de notre existence, et de son échéance mortelle, nous incite à vivre pleinement. Pour cela nous choisissons, autant que possible, notre profession, nos loisirs, nos amis, notre cadre de vie et nos options religieuses ou politiques. Nous devons pouvoir choisir aussi les conditions dans lesquelles, un jour, cette vie bien remplie s'arrêtera.

Parce qu'ils n'ont pas fait ce choix, et parce qu'on refuse d'abréger leurs souffrances au nom d'une prétendue morale, des malades incurables, des infirmes, sont condamnés à subir une 'pseudo-vie' jusqu'à son terme 'naturel', quel que soit leur état mental et physique.

Je suis de ceux qui souhaitent mourir dans la dignité et je partage tout à fait les convictions des adhérents de l'Association pour le Droit de Mourir dans la Dignité qui apporte son aide aux malades opposés à toutes les formes d'acharnement thérapeutique, ainsi qu'à leur famille. Loin de pousser au suicide, les adhérents sont inspirés par l'amour de la vie, dont la mort est le dernier acte. Ils veulent le préparer, pour qu'on ne prolonge en aucun cas une vie qui ne serait plus que déchéance. L'important, pour moi, est d'accorder à ceux qui en expriment clairement le désir un moyen de mettre un terme à leur vie de façon digne.

Unit 6. La Pollution

'Les pays occidentaux doivent absolument limiter la place de l'automobile s'ils ne veulent pas se détruire.'

Relevez dans le texte des exemples qui justifient ce point de vue et donnez en français vos réactions personnelles. N'oubliez pas d'utliser des mots de liaison.

Écrivez un maximum de 300 mots.

Des milliers de personnes, dans les grandes villes occidentales, meurent chaque année de maladies respiratoires, ou de cancers, dus à la mauvaise qualité de l'air pollué par l'automobile. Les responsables sont dénoncés: transporteurs routiers, constructeurs automobiles, bétonneurs…

Pourtant, il me paraît indispensable de tirer la sonnette d'alarme pour inciter à plus de prudence comportementale de la part des citoyens. Aux dernières nouvelles, les politiques et les lobbies financiers s'efforceraient désormais de limiter les dégâts: pour relier la ville et la banlieue, on voit se développer les réseaux de transports collectifs: des tramways sont créés (ou recréés), parfois même dans des villes déjà pourvues du métro, pour inciter les automobilistes à laisser leur voiture au garage. De même, certaines agglomérations s'équipent de voitures et de vélos électriques (non polluants) de location. Mais la prise de conscience des citoyens eux-mêmes est-elle bien réelle?

Je dois avouer qu'il ne me paraît ni réaliste, ni envisageable de vouloir ramener dans les villes ceux qui ont fait le libre choix de s'en éloigner pour vivre différemment. Pour ma part, je ne vois pas pourquoi les gens renonceraient au plaisir de mettre de la distance entre 'bureau et dodo' afin de retrouver un pavillon avec jardin après une journée de stress en ville! Par contre, j'estime qu'il faut absolument faire de la réclame pour le co-voiturage, jusqu'à ce qu'il soit couramment pratiqué. Quant au réseau ferroviaire, s'il offrait un service irréprochable il permettrait de réduire considérablement l'utilisation des automobiles particulières.

Il est encourageant de noter que, partout où ces efforts sont réalisés, les observatoires de surveillance de la pollution enregistrent une amélioration notable de la qualité de l'air. Alors, luttons tous pour faire respirer la ville!

JENNY OLLERENSHAW © 1998, 2002

Unit 7. L'Association Emmaüs

'Les exclus ont autant besoin de dignité, de reconnaissance sociale et de considération que d'un logement, d'un travail et d'une formation.'

Relevez dans le texte des exemples qui soutiennent ce point de vue et donnez en français vos réactions personnelles.

Écrivez un maximum de 250 mots.

Ecouter, accompagner, aider les exclus sans les assister: tel est le sens de la mission des salariés et bénévoles de l'Association Emmaüs fondée en 1949 par l'abbé Pierre.

Centres d'accueil ouverts à chaque homme ou femme 'sans toit, sans droits, sans emploi', les Communautés leur permettent de reprendre espoir et de redonner un sens à leur vie. Imprégné de sa foi et d'un profond respect de la personne humaine, l'abbé Pierre a su mobiliser les bonnes volontés, intervenir auprès des responsables politiques, quand et où il le fallait, pour expliquer inlassablement que l'homme a tout autant besoin d'amour que de pain.

Je suis convaincu(e) que le regard d'amitié que l'on portera à une personne qui souffre d'être rejetée, marginalisée, est aussi important que la nourriture ou le lit qu'on lui attribuera dans un centre d'accueil. Il faut savoir passer du temps avec un être qui souffre pour essayer de mieux le connaître, pour l'aider à trouver du travail, à suivre une formation, et surtout pour lui montrer qu'il n'a pas perdu sa dignité.

Parce qu'elle fait tout cela, l'Association Emmaüs m'apparaît comme un modèle, car elle est à la fois une association caritative (comme bien d'autres tout aussi méritantes) mais également une institution reconnue, capable de faire pression auprès des pouvoirs publics pour défendre les plus démunis, forte de son bon droit et du soutien de tous les hommes de bien.

Unit 8. Le Chômage et le Racisme

'Le «Front National» a tort de dire que les immigrés sont responsables du chômage en France.'

Relevez dans le texte des arguments qui justifient ce point de vue et donnez en français vos réactions personnelles. N'oubliez pas d'utliser des mots de liaison là où il convient.

Écrivez un maximum de 320 mots.

Le 'Front National' affirme que les immigrés seraient des voleurs d'emplois, tous responsables du chômage en France. Or, dire qu'il y a trois millions d'immigrés en France, et donc autant de chômeurs me paraît loin d'être exact.

Tout d'abord, il faut s'entendre sur la définition du mot 'immigré'. Pour commencer, parmi ces 'immigrés', seraient notamment recensées un grand nombre de personnes devenues françaises car naturalisées. De plus, le FN emploie ce mot pour se référer aux ressortissants non-européens. Or ceux-ci ne représentent qu'une partie des 3,6 millions d'étrangers vivant en France. Finalement, quand on parle de chômage, on considère la population active, et non pas les enfants, qui ne prennent le travail de personne. Au bout du compte, les étrangers actifs non-européens représentent moins d'un quart de la population étrangère.

À cela il faut ajouter que seulement trois Français sur dix accepteraient le genre d'emploi proposés aux immigrés. Les statistiques indiquent également que, globalement, les étrangers sont plus touchés par le chômage (18,6%) que les Français (9,5%). Mais si le FN déclare que 'les immigrés profitent du chômage' à travers les 'mécanismes sociaux protecteurs', il faut corriger ce genre d'allégations: l'allocation chômage ne peut être accordée qu'aux personnes justifiant qu'elles ont effectivement travaillé et cotisé auprès des organismes sociaux pendant plusieurs mois de façon continue.